OUTOFSHAPEWORTHLESSLOSER

OUTOFSHAPEWORTHLESSLOSER

A MEMOIR OF FIGURE SKATING, F*CKING UP, AND FIGURING IT OUT

GRACIE GOLD

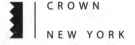

CROWN
NEW YORK

OUTOFSHAPEWORTHLESSLOSER

Published in the United States by Crown, an imprint of the Crown Publishing
Group, a division of Penguin Random House LLC, New York.

CROWN and the Crown colophon are registered trademarks
of Penguin Random House LLC.

Library of Congress Cataloging-in-Publication Data
Names: Gold, Gracie, 1995– author.
Title: Outofshapeworthlessloser / Gracie Gold.
Other titles: Out of shape worthless loser
Description: First edition. | New York: Crown, [2024]
Identifiers: LCCN 2023048670 (print) | LCCN 2023048671 (ebook) |
ISBN 9780593444047 (hardcover) | ISBN 9780593444054 (ebook)
Subjects: LCSH: Gold, Gracie, 1995– | Figure skaters—United States—
Biography. | Women Olympic athletes—United States—Biography. | Eating
disorders in women—United States. | Women—United States—Social aspects.
Classification: LCC GV850.G65 A3 2024 (print) | LCC GV850.G65 (ebook) |
DDC 796.91/2092 [B]—dc23/eng/20231101
LC record available at https://lccn.loc.gov/2023048670
LC ebook record available at https://lccn.loc.gov/2023048671

Printed in the United States of America on acid-free paper

crownpublishing.com

1 3 5 7 9 8 6 4 2

First Edition

Book design by Caroline Cunningham

To Carly, the best parts of this book, my life,

and myself are all because of you.

To everyone who's ever thought the world might be better off

without them, it's not. This is for the people who stayed

and the ones who couldn't.

CONTENTS

I do not at all understand the mystery of grace—only

that it meets us where we are

but does not leave us where it found us.

—Anne Lamott

AUTHOR'S NOTE

Putting my story down in writing was my way of processing a journey that has encompassed the highest of highs and the lowest of lows. I've done my best to be factual and fair in my recounting of the people and events that shaped my skating and how those people and events impacted my life. I have changed some names to keep the focus on my experience—and on the change I'd like to make in a system rigged toward those with the power to silence others. My perspective is my own, shaped inexorably by my struggles with depression, anxiety, disordered eating, and traumas, including sexual assault and suicidal ideation, that are described in these pages. I can appreciate how, the more you can relate to any of these subjects, the harder the book you hold in your hands might be to read. If that's the case, please proceed with caution, care, and self-compassion.

OUTOFSHAPEWORTHLESSLOSER

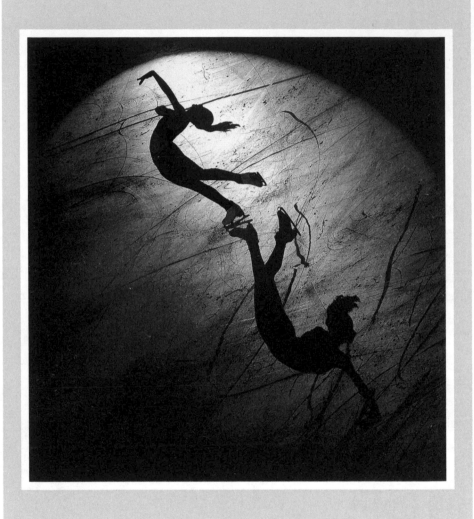

PROLOGUE

My days were meant to be filled with polishing my programs for the upcoming Winter Olympics, wrapping up interviews with the national and international media, and awaiting the television rollout of Olympic promotional spots that I had already starred in. Instead, I was in a recovery center surrounded by heroin addicts and meth users and self-harmers.

I was just starting to process how my career as an Olympic figure skater had turned me into a bright, shiny object to be gazed at and admired, only to shatter me in the process. In the communal area of a dorm best described as motor inn chic, I stared at my newest assignment: Write a letter to my addictions.

September 2017

Dear Skating,

I am writing to you because I cannot decide if I hate you or if I love you. You are a part of me—my identifier to the world. You are my esteem, my joy, my sense of self all tied up in one. I hate you—but I cannot leave you. I was so excited to meet you. Just one lap around the rink and I was home. You made me feel special. Some people even said that you made me extraordinary.

You've brought me to places I never dreamed of.

But you were a double-sided coin.

You've brought me across the world, you've brought me so much passion and love, you've introduced me to the most amazing people. You've exposed me to once-in-a-lifetime opportunities. I flourished under your guidance and love. But I also was crushed by the weight of your expectations.

I abused your love and became addicted to your rush. I watched as you ripped apart my family and others, destroyed my life, and brought me to lows I didn't know were possible. You are the mask I wear the most. Who am I under it? I have no idea. It's time to say goodbye to this relationship. My toxic shame spiral will continue no more. I will not let you ruin my life. For what? More medals? Fame? Money?

I've come to realize I am exceptional with or without you. You introduced me to an eating disorder, alcohol, depression, anxiety, and perfectionism. The combination almost killed me. I wanted it to kill me. But now I am awake. I am alive and do not need you. You are no longer the only facet of my life. You're just a tiny carat on the beautiful diamond ring that is my life now. I can't imagine my life without you—but I'm going to try.

Goodbye, my dear friend,

xoG

A handwriting analyst might have concluded from the paragraphs of left-slanting letters that my childhood had left me severely emotionally repressed. "Exquisitely trained" is the preferred wording in the skating world. Over many years I had been painstakingly conditioned to make people feel something when I was on the ice, but to do that required stuffing down my own emotions.

I can't do that anymore. And I won't.

ACCESSORIZING THE TRUTH

It's so on-brand that my skating origin story, the one that I've recited more than the Pledge of Allegiance, is a fabrication, a tale spun from granules of truth into an easily digestible cotton-candy anecdote. But if I'm going to offer up the truth of my life now, I can't approach this as I did too many failed triple jumps over the years: nervous and afraid of looking bad. I've committed to telling every last part, no matter how anxious it makes me (I can feel a neck rash forming already).

I might as well start from the beginning, with the story that I've always told: A boy in my class invited me to his birthday party at a sparkling new rink in Springfield, Missouri, shortly before I turned eight. That much is true. But when I laced up my rental boots and jumped on the ice, it wasn't my first time on skates, as I've made it sound in the past. I had teetered as a two-year-old on a frozen pond near our house when we were living in Massachusetts. That experience was a nightmare, reducing me to a shivering puddle of tears.

But a few years later, I was in my element in the music box that was Springfield's Jordan Valley Ice Park rink, which pulsed with pop hits like Justin Timberlake's "Rock Your Body." Given the town's conservatism, it was like having bootleg music flow from the speakers. The Springfield of my youth was the kind of place where dinner at a friend's house was preceded by everyone joining hands in a circle and singing "God Bless America." The rink offered me an alternative world, one that paired the freedom of movement, including flight, with shocking lyrics like "Just wanna rock you girl / I'll have whatever you have / Come on, just give it a whirl."

The story that I told for years was that on my way out of the rink that day I picked up a flyer advertising skating lessons and begged my mom to sign me up. Yeah, no. The flyer that caught my eye was for hockey lessons. I was rough-and-tumble. My best friends were almost exclusively boys. I wanted to chase the puck, not perfection, on the ice.

But hockey lessons were a nonstarter for my mom, who shuddered at the thought of the aggressions that I might unleash with a stick in my hand. She and my father often told the story of how, when I was six or seven and playing soccer on a coed team, I ran neck and neck with a boy who positioned himself between me and the loose ball. I whacked him across the face with my arm to knock him out of the way and got my foot on the ball first, but my triumph was short-lived. The boy sobbed and I received a red card from the referee, resulting in an automatic ejection. I couldn't help but detect a note of pride in my parents' voices every time they trotted this story out at parties. My competitiveness was something that could set me apart if it was channeled correctly. On the drive home, I asked Mom why I had been pulled from the game, because I honestly had no idea. She took her eyes off the road long enough to swivel her head to stare at me. "Gracie, you punched a boy," she said. "You cannot do that!"

So, yes, skating lessons struck my mother as the preferable option. It was a competitive outlet that seemed safe. Respectable, even. Gracie Goon was not a persona she wished to encourage. I became a figure skater because those sparkly, sequined dresses offered camouflage for my inner tomboy and cover for my impulse control issues. On the ice, the only person I could hurt was myself.

So completely did I internalize my sanitized origin story that my recollections of that soccer game—indeed, of my life before the birthday skating party—are foggy. That hockey story, for example, had completely slipped my mind until my mom brought it up recently in a conversation.

If it's hard for me to keep track of what's real and what's fake, it's because figure skating has split me into three people. There's my public self, Gracie Gold, an Olympic bronze medalist and two-time national champion who wore designer costumes and drew comparisons to Grace Kelly with her platinum-blond bun and carefully applied mask of mascara, red lipstick, and a permafrost smile. There's my private self, Grace Elizabeth, an artsy eccentric who lives in baggy sweatpants and oversized sweatshirts and sneakers with no socks, crochets granny hats and scarves in her free time, wears no makeup, and never leaves home without her vape. Then there's my secret self, Outofshapeworthlessloser, a judgmental perfectionist whose self-destructive tendencies nearly killed me.

Throughout my life, each of these personas has dominated at different times. This memoir is my attempt to reconcile these selves into a single being. She might be messy. But at least she'll be Me.

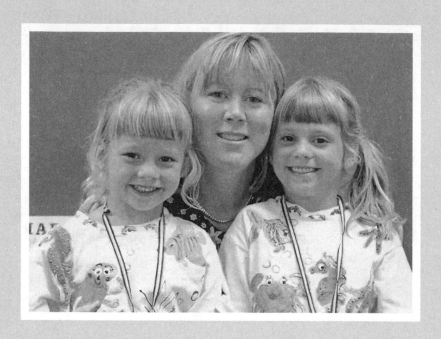

GRACE ELIZABETH

PART ONE

But it's no use going back to yesterday, because
I was a different person then.

—Lewis Carroll, *Alice's Adventures
in Wonderland*

1

PERFECT OBSESSION

My compulsion for order revealed itself early. As soon as I was old enough to reach the hangers in my closet, I arranged my clothing by color. Strangely, red and white mixed together in any other context forms my favorite color, pink. But in my bedroom, their careless converging created meltdown-level angst.

Which made me an ideal mark for skating. I'm a big believer that sports choose you rather than the other way around. I dabbled in enough of them to know: soccer, swimming, gymnastics, dance. None suited my temperament as well as skating did, but my time spent in the other activities wasn't wasted. Along the way I developed strength, flexibility, self-confidence, and spatial awareness, all of which would facilitate my success in skating. The discomfort I had felt on the ice as a toddler was long gone by age eight, replaced by an athleticism that made me feel all-powerful in my body and convinced there was nothing I couldn't do.

Perfection seemed not just possible but, with enough practice, a reasonable goal. That was reassuring because from as far back as I can remember, I hated to make a mistake. Could. Not. Stand.

It. If I misspelled one word on a homework assignment, I'd furiously erase the whole sentence and start over. You don't want to know how many times I've reworked this chapter.

Skating, with its emphasis on precision and perfection, was the ideal obsession for me. It held my attention much more than swimming, with its black-lined sensory deprivation tank. And it didn't scare me like gymnastics. I loved running full speed toward the vault and launching myself skyward, but I feared the balance beam. My discomfort at being suspended like a tightrope walker was acute. I wanted to feel more grounded before flinging myself in the air (it didn't help that the leotards were so itchy they made me want to jump out of my skin). Of course, there were times when skating scared me, too, but the difficulty of the skills increased so gradually, like water coming to a slow boil, that I was never really conscious of it until the spills that were once no big deal were suddenly resulting in bone bruises and fractures. The anxiety, the apprehension, the pain—they rose in lockstep with my skill level and expectations.

Nobody expected much of me when I participated in an ice show at the end of my introductory lessons. It was 2003 and skating was riding a wave of popularity in the United States. Sarah Hughes and Michelle Kwan had made the podium at the last Olympics (with Sasha Cohen behind Michelle in fourth), and Michelle was the reigning women's world champion. Skating was near the height of its appeal in the United States, but in Springfield it had yet to catch fire. As I recall, there were fewer than six students, all girls, in my group lessons. Its lack of a coolness factor in Springfield matched my own nerdiness, which was part of its initial appeal. I liked that I was doing something that most people couldn't or wouldn't try. It suited me just fine that I didn't have to share the ice with a lot of people—including, at first, my fraternal twin sister, Carly.

My sister and I did most things together, but figure skating was the first endeavor that was mine alone. I was very possessive about it, referring to it as "my Saturday activity." That would change after Carly gave up riding horses, which had been *her* Saturday activity, to join me at the rink. Surprisingly, I didn't mind sharing skating with Carly as much as I thought I would, because from day one she's been my main source of comfort and security. Ten years later, our father would tell a *New York Post* reporter that he and Mom were torn about how much to push us, saying there was "a lot of wailing and gnashing our teeth." But in the beginning skating was bliss. Twice a week, Mom dropped us off at the rink, waved goodbye, and said, "Have fun!"

An unexpected perk of skating was that it—at least at first—brought me closer to my mom, a girly-girl gifted with twin tomboys whom she loved and supported even though we often must have seemed inscrutable to her. Denise Gold grew up near San Diego, California. She liked to skateboard and roller-skate and would later play recreational tennis, but sunbathing was my mom's main jam as a kid.

The female-centric sport of skating opened a whole new world to me. It was my initiation into a sparkly culture of shiny stones—skating-speak for beads—and glamorous dresses. Mom was thrilled to serve as my guide. We bonded over the outfits that she helped me pick out for lessons and then competitions. I can remember us pawing through the clothes racks and Mom's face lighting up: "Isn't this cute? This is so cute! I love this!" I became a dress-up doll that my mom loved to clothe in pretty costumes, including many that she sewed herself.

I was proud to have the cool mom, someone who found a way to feed her artistic side while carrying out the prosaic duties of parenting. She'd make many of our clothes because of her love of design, rather than out of necessity. Her attitude was, basically, why buy something new when you can make something unique? She applied the same approach to furnishing our homes, filling them with thrift-store furniture that she artistically restored.

I still have vivid pictures in my head of some of the dresses she made for me. They were pieced together with such care and creativity. I remember an outfit that Mom made from scratch using yellow and white bugle beads that she individually stitched by hand onto the dress (because I was skating to the instrumental song "Popcorn," duh!). Despite the labor involved, she did not skimp on the bugle beads. It was so cute. There was one problem she hadn't anticipated. All those beads made the costume incredibly heavy. It bent the metal hanger that held it, which should have been our first clue that it was going to be less than ideal to skate in. I might as well have been skating in a wet fur coat. I have no idea what happened to that dress. I wish I'd kept it. It rivaled any of the beautiful pieces that designers Brad Griffies and Josiane Lamond, she of my famous *Firebird* costume, would create for me in the future.

At the time, though, I probably expressed ambivalence about it. With the benefit of time and distance, I can see how lucky I was to wear Mom's unique creations. But my elementary and middle school selves gravitated toward conformity. Especially in the conservative Midwest, where I spent those years, happiness was equated with maintaining appearances; of coming across as pious and picture-perfect.

Everything about our family's existence, from the tidy neighborhood and the backyard pool to the riding and skating lessons, screamed respectability. My dad, an anesthesiologist, and my mother, a retired emergency room nurse, were self-made successes, *The Official Preppy Handbook*–toting believers in the American dream. In an interview with the Springfield, Illinois, *State Journal-Register*, my dad painted this family portrait: "I

challenge anyone to imagine a Midwest family, very humble beginnings, small-town, rural Missouri, small-town Illinois, just
doing something on a daily basis, day in, day out, working hard."

The skating world reinforced conventional norms. I quickly
picked up on how Mom's costumes, no matter how clever and
well-constructed, were met by disapproving looks from coaches
and judges. I intuited their judgment and pushed back on Mom's
inventions. I wanted my outfits to look like everyone else's. I remember begging her for the costumes hanging on the racks. I
was such a shit. Bless my mom for not taking it personally. In
fact, I think she was secretly relieved: *You don't like all that hand-
beading that took me hours to complete? Fine!*

I was surprised to discover that I enjoyed playing dress-up.
Who knew that a budding femininity was buried beneath the
flannel shirts and oversized hoodies and baggy sweatpants that
made up my day-to-day wardrobe? But going glamorous had its
downsides, too. I struggled with the body-hugging contours of
costumes and the accompanying tights, which exacerbated an
extreme sensory sensitivity that my loose-fitting clothing helped
me manage. I'd never be caught dead wearing Mickey Mouse
ears, but I'd find them far more tolerable than anything with
seams, socks included. I've skated sockless on and off over the
years because I couldn't find a pair of socks that didn't make my
skin feel like it was covered in mosquito bites. (I.T.C.H.: It's the
cross-stitching, honey.) Same with denim jeans, which were a
nonstarter for me because the seams felt like knives on my skin.
Whoever came up with the idea for jeggings deserves the Nobel
Peace Prize for stopping the fighting in our house. Jeggings allowed my mom and me to establish a truce in our wardrobe wars.
I could wear them without wanting to scratch my skin till it bled.

When it came to the tights that skating required, only one
brand, Nita Sports, was soft and buttery smooth enough. The tag-

less label was key. One time, we showed up for an ice show and Mom had packed a brand of tights that itched. I burst into tears and informed her that under no circumstances could I wear them. I was inconsolable. She said she was sorry that she had messed up but I had no choice. I had to skate in the torturous tights. It would be a test of how well I could cope with discomfort, she said. People were counting on me. I couldn't let them down. Mom framed it as a learning moment. If I couldn't figure out how to regulate my emotions, she said, I was destined for a difficult life.

Despite my costume issues, I loved the attention that skating gave me (as befits someone born under the Leo astrological sign). Skating made me feel special—at least in the beginning. I was nine years old the first time I can recall seeing my name in the newspaper. The *Springfield News-Leader* in Missouri reported on my victory at a competition in Kansas City in its June 17, 2005, edition. I was still representing the Jordan Valley Figure Skating Club, but I would soon outgrow my coaches there.

The difficulty of the sport, especially for beginners, did not slow me in the least. I loved the challenge. *Fun fact:* A figure skating blade is about three-sixteenths of an inch wide, with two edges that you lean on to glide around on. The more you lean in to the edges, the more points you can accrue, but only to a degree. Lean in too far or hit a rut in the ice and you'll fall, surrendering more points than if you had played it safe. It's an unsubtle metaphor. I would basically spend my whole career pushing it as far as I could, for as long as I could, and fail many, many times before I succeeded.

Strangely, it didn't bother me to fall. There are kids I come across now in my clinics who'll do jumps with little air under them or stick to the jump they know they can land cleanly rather than risk me seeing them take a tumble on the ice. I don't understand voluntarily clipping your wings. For me, there's nothing cooler than the sensation of soaring through the air. It's addictive—worth the possibility of a crash landing.

Another thing I loved about skating was that there existed a methodical system for learning and advancement. There were so many fun skills to learn. From my first swizzle, people gushed to my mom about my athleticism. Bunny hops, crossovers, spins— I picked up the basic skills with ease. My mother was encouraged to bring me to the rink for private lessons, which sometimes required me to rise before the sun. She didn't blink. She just herded me into the car and turned on the engine. Her life philosophy, which she applied to her parenting, is that everything you do, you do to the max. To this day, I can hear her voice in my head: *To the max, Gracie!*

In the beginning, there was no expectation that I'd ever approach anywhere near the level of my idol, Michelle Kwan. Mom was happy to indulge my skating mostly because all that spinning and jumping and gliding had a tranquilizing effect on me. She was relieved to stumble upon what appeared to be a healthy outlet for my high-strung personality, my impulsivity, my perfectionism. If she had only known what we know now.

I was a relative latecomer to the sport, but I didn't know it until I started to venture outside Missouri for events and interacted with skaters my age who had been on the ice for half their lives. A few were already being homeschooled to accommodate the sport's demands. My parents couldn't wrap their heads around the idea of families arranging their days to accommodate a grade-schooler's skating. That was never going to be me and Carly, they said.

Nothing was more important to my parents than academics. I

was an adult before I realized that there were people who failed classes. I couldn't conceive of "earning" a C or D, much less an F. I recall getting one B in all my years of school, in high school biology, and I thought it was the end of the world.

I was a fast learner in skating, which enabled me to catch up quickly. I'll never forget the first time I launched my body into the air and landed my first Axel—a one-and-a-half-revolution jump that's a key milestone for young skaters. It was awkward but I stayed upright. I was nine years old and my coaches at the Springfield, Missouri, rink were incredulous. They fawned over me like I was a rock star. I can't deny that my love for the sport was tangled up with my mastery of it. But was I good enough to one day skate in the Olympics?

Nobody could have predicted it. The odds were stacked against me despite all my built-in advantages: my obsession with single, repetitive tasks; my natural coordination; my flair for the dramatic; my conventionally attractive looks; and, last but certainly not least, my father's anesthesiologist's salary, enough to cover equipment and coaching, which are not cheap.

I always thought it was so cute when people thought that I was a prodigy along the lines of Nathan Chen, who at age eight was landing clean double combinations. Unlike Nathan, I did not explode on the scene like fireworks. Other skaters had started before me and had a head start. I was the overnight sensation several years in the making.

The ladder of progression in skating has changed somewhat since the 2020 pandemic, but when I was coming up, it consisted of the following rungs: basic skills, pre-preliminary, preliminary, pre-juvenile, juvenile, intermediate, novice, junior, and senior. So, yeah, a lot of steps in this stairway to glory. At each level, the fields at nationals are typically filled by skaters who have survived and advanced through two rounds of qualifying competitions called regionals and sectionals.

Given how much I love going my own way, you'd think my first taste of national skating success would have been in singles. But it was actually as a pairs skater. In 2007, I finished seventh at the U.S. Junior Figure Skating Championship with Sean Hickey, whose mother coached us. Sean and I were decent freestyle skaters and our side-by-side double Lutz–double toe combination set us apart. We performed lifts, just not overhead ones, and we had a throw Axel in our repertoire that was so much fun to do. I enjoyed getting tossed in the air. I liked that it was more acrobatic than singles. It was my dream to go all the way to the top in pairs. Singles was fine, but pairs was where it was at as far as I was concerned. As I remember it, though, Sean broke his arm in a non-skating mishap and then started high school, and his interest in the sport waned.

After our partnership ended, I was flown to Los Angeles for pairs tryouts like I was a kid actor auditioning to be a Mouseketeer or something, but ultimately it didn't work out. The logistics didn't make sense. I'd have had to move to Los Angeles with Mom, and Carly would have had to stay behind with Dad, which we decided would have made us all miserable. It was a hard pass then. It wouldn't be later. But at age eleven, the thought of our family living apart was unfathomable to us. The concept of breaking up the Golds for something as frivolous as figure skating violated the Midwest social contract that put God and family first. Not to mention that it would have shattered the united family image that we labored to maintain.

I still was leading what I'd consider a conventional childhood. I had non-skating friends at school: boys I liked to play kickball, dodgeball, tetherball, or soccer with at recess, and girls I liked to sit on the swings and gossip with. I spent a lot of time outdoors when I wasn't at the rink but I still found time to read books I checked out from the library or do puzzles or play board games like Scattergories with Carly and our parents. As a family, we went to the movies on weekends and ate out every Saturday.

The first real accommodation we made for skating happened when I was nine or ten and we began making a three-hundred-mile drive every Friday to work with a woman in Springfield, Illinois, who came recommended by my coaches in Missouri. Mom didn't mind making the drive because she recognized that to keep improving I really did need to "step it up," as she put it. Our Suburban SUV had three rows of seats, so Carly and I would each spread out in a single row and sleep, watch DVDs, or do homework during the long drive. The miles on the odometer piled up and so did the truancy letters from our school district for all the class time we were missing. I didn't know then that my parents had their own reasons for wanting to spend all that time apart. But they also were flattered when people praised my potential and undaunted by the commitment required of all of us to squeeze the most out of this gift that I had been given.

I have few fond memories of this coach—let's call her Cruella—who aggressively played favorites and pitted skaters against one another. One of us would be on the ice running through our program and Cruella would say, loud enough for everyone to hear, "She sounds like a hippo out there. Thud. Thud. Thud." The girls being criticized were as young as eight.

Cruella disallowed the wearing of pants or leggings during training—dresses and tights only, ladies!—and bestowed skating dresses, made by her, on us to wear on special occasions, or to mark milestones, like landing a clean double Axel. If there was no ice availability at our regular rink, Cruella would drive us to another town and book us into hotel rooms sans parents. If a skater was visiting from out of town, they would stay at Cruella's home.

On occasion she would invite all her students to spend the night. The sleepovers were presented to us as treats, a reward for our hard training. To the best of my knowledge, nothing physically or sexually inappropriate happened at these get-togethers. But that does not mean there wasn't something *off* about them.

My mother definitely had misgivings about the gatherings but broke down and let us attend one after Carly and I begged and begged her to let us go. She arrived early the next morning to collect us. We didn't speak of the experience.

I vaguely recall that one of the other skaters essentially became Cruella's charge. Her parents lived in another town and signed off on Cruella becoming her legal guardian. And if my memory serves, she wasn't the only one. It flabbergasts me that adults were willing to cede their authority to her, as so many did. Were they naive? Happy to outsource their parenting? In thrall to their child's potential? Blinded by their own ambitions for their child?

All of us, the adults included, were marionettes and Cruella was pulling the strings. She chose our music. She cut the tracks. She choreographed. She coached. She screamed. When Cruella aimed her ire at Carly, my sister would shrink into the background or cry, not because she was scared or upset but as her coping mechanism. When Cruella lashed out at me, I lashed back louder. Anger was my protection. It got back to me years later that Cruella told people she had always known I'd become a star. I call bullshit! She was always doing her best to humiliate me. Or maybe she didn't like me because I stood up to her.

Children are perfectly capable of identifying a schoolyard bully in a grown-up's body. They may not respect them, but because of the power coaches wield, they'll listen to them and do as they say. The years I spent with Cruella normalized the kind of controlling behavior that, even if it produces positive results on the ice, can be ruinous to a child's personal development. I look back at this period of my life and wonder, was it a fever dream? It was so weird in so many respects, but at the time we simply arched our (already) professionally waxed eyebrows and carried on.

I was working with Cruella when I conducted my first newspaper interviews. My mom sat in on them, but not to make sure I said everything "correctly" or "perfectly." She was there to rein me in if I started speaking without running my words through my brain's filter first, because when I was little, especially, I was prone to blurting out the first thing that popped into my head. Her direction, however gentle, did play a role in choreographing my origin story. I mentioned the birthday party, and as I recall, my mom took it from there. "Gracie saw girls spinning on the ice," she said, "and she wanted to learn how to do that." As time went on, I added my own twists. "While I circled around and around in my brown rental skates, I studied a group of skaters spinning in the center," I later told the Olympic media in 2014. "I was fascinated! When my mom picked me up, I began a campaign for skating lessons."

Gracie Goon, the would-be hockey player, was gone, erased to make room for the Disney princess version that hewed more closely to the wholesome-girl-next-door script.

It was fitting because my whole world as a child was a stage. Even my home was its own movie set, with each room carefully curated by my mom to embody a theme. Consider my childhood bedroom. The walls were painted my favorite color, pink, with a border trim that featured pink bows. Using stencils, my mom painted fairies on the walls. My nightstand was a piece she found at a thrift shop, sanded, and painted pink. By hand, she made a pink tulle canopy, with bows, for my bed and found a duvet and sheets to match. She put considerable time and thought into making the kind of cozy home that she wished she had had as a child.

In many ways, my childhood home was the ideal environment for nurturing a champion skater—at least until my family's secrets brought down the whole production. I learned at a young age how to smile when I felt like crying.

2

GROWING UP GOLD

When I look back at my struggles now and search for the red flags I should have seen, the exact moment when I went off the rails, it would be easy for me to point to people like my coach, Cruella—those who transformed skating from something fun into something toxic. But if I'm being honest with myself, I have to start much earlier, because the conditions that would later contribute to my high-profile crash and burn had already been established on the day I was born.

Twins are notorious for being born weeks ahead of schedule. Not us. Carly and I arrived in August 1995 several days past our due date and some forty minutes apart, establishing from the very beginning a pattern of lateness that I've never been able to break. I call it GST (Gracie Standard Time), and it is reliably fifteen minutes behind schedule. I weighed eight pounds and Carly weighed seven. I can't imagine what it must have been like those last few weeks to be our mother, who was forty-one at the time and precariously balancing two hundred pounds on her five-foot frame. It wasn't just our late arrivals and natural births that tested Mom's mettle. She went through hell to conceive us. After years of futility, she used in-vitro fertilization. For that, I'm in awe of her. These days, my mom and I have a complicated relationship, but I can't deny that her strength is impressive. When I think of the phrase "whiskey in a teacup," I picture her.

According to Dad, Mom was supposed to have labor induced on the sixteenth of August. But early that morning she was contacted by her doctor, who said there was no room at the maternity ward. Every bed was taken. As annoyed as she was to have to wait another day, there was a bright side. We wouldn't be born as *Wednesday's children full of woe,* to paraphrase the Old English nursery rhyme. Full of woe, no. We were Thursday babies. *Thursday's child has far to go.*

I showed a flair for the dramatic from the start. An ultrasound taken by the doctor to confirm our positions for delivery revealed that I was feet-first. The doctor was preparing Mom for a C-section when I somehow turned myself around so that I was head-down and ready for my grand entrance. I'm not surprised that I maneuvered myself in the birth canal so that I beat Carly to meet our parents. I can totally imagine it: me elbowing my way into the lead, just as I later would on the soccer field, establishing at the beginning of our lives the pattern from which we've only recently deviated: me fearlessly forging ahead, testing the waters, while my sister holds back, carefully weighing her options before joining me. According to family lore, I came out screaming bloody murder. Carly, on the other hand, was as quiet as dawn. When she was placed on Mom's chest, the nurses remarked on how her eyes held wisdom. In our first hour in this world, our roles were assigned. Carly was the wise one. I was the spitfire.

Sometimes when I tell the story of our delivery, I leave out the part about the sizable gap between my arrival and Carly's, because when I remain faithful to the script people invariably have a lightbulb moment. They go, "Oh my God, your mom didn't have a C-section? She gave birth vaginally?" I don't know about you, but the less I'm drawn into any discussion of my mom's vagina, the better.

Temperamentally, Carly and I could not be more different. Mom used to laugh at teachers who suggested separating us in school so that we could forge our own identities. "Trust me," she'd say. "They may be twins, but they are two distinct people." She wasn't wrong. Our dissimilar dispositions were on full display in Mrs. V.'s first-grade class in Texas. Carly has always been adept at sizing up adults and assessing what's required of her to stay in their good graces. I believe the term for it is "people pleaser."

I was the opposite. Social nuances for me as a child were like dirty jokes. They went right over my head, which is why I thought nothing of writing in an assigned journal: "Mrs. V. is a fun sucker. She sucks the fun out of learning." So lacking in self-awareness was I, it never occurred to me that Mrs. V. might read my words. I simply emptied my heart out onto the page. That entry led to an awkward conversation at the next parent-teacher conference. I remember Mom coming home and saying, "Really, Gracie? Mrs. V. sucks the fun out of learning? What were you thinking?" Later in the year, when Mrs. V. assigned us to interview an adult we admire and write a one-page report, Mom saw an opportunity for me to redeem myself. She suggested that I interview Mrs. V., then sat in on my Q&A with her. I sweetly asked Mrs. V. what made her become a teacher and she said that in her day women could be nurses or teachers and since she hated the sight of blood, she became a teacher. I glanced at my mom and the look on her face was like, *Hmmm, maybe Gracie has a point.*

I had no filter. Anything I thought or felt, I expressed. Not for nothing, Mom's pet names for us were Grace Storm Cloud and Carly Sunshine.

No question, I could be a handful. When Mom was pregnant, she received identical baby blankets from a friend as a shower gift. They were arranged neatly in our cribs when Mom and Dad brought us home from the hospital. The blankets were composed of different squares. In the center was one with a bunny holding three balloons: blue, pink, and yellow. I loved Blankie, as I called mine. I took it everywhere, which is how I came to leave it at a sleepover hosted by a friend whose family moved the next day, before I could get Blankie back. I was inconsolable. I sobbed for two days straight. Carly couldn't stand to see me upset, so she offered me her blanket. I still have it. In twenty-eight years, I've spent less than a week of nights without it. I'm so attached to Blankie, if I go out for drinks with friends, I'll throw him in the back of the car just in case I end up sleeping over at someone's place. Make of it what you will that I rely on a comfort object from early childhood to feel safe and secure as an adult.

It was so on-brand for Carly to give up her blanket for me. She has consistently put my needs ahead of hers over the years. And how do I repay her? Rarely in kind. I remember when we were relatively new to skating and acquired Züca customized roller bags. With their array of colors and built-in seats and wheels that lit up as they went round and round, the bags were as coveted at the rink as Birkin bags in other cliques. One morning after a skating session, Carly rolled hers to the back of our Suburban and left it next to the open hatch, assuming I'd toss it in with my own. Call it a moment of mischievousness or straight-out spite, but my child brain thought it would be hilarious if I deposited my bag in the rear and left hers where it was. While backing up, Mom ran over it. Crunch. The bag's metal frame got stuck against the wheel well and lifted the car like a jacking device. We had to call a towing service to get Carly's bag extricated from the wheel. I remember we were over an hour late to school that day. But on the bright side, Carly's skates miraculously survived unscathed.

Carly and I relate a lot to Athena and Nike. Carly is Athena, our family's goddess of wisdom, and I'm Nike, goddess of victory. We're pretty much joined at the hip, as were they, and even though Carly wasn't buzzing around the battlefield like I was, she was pulling her own weight in other ways. Of the two of us, Carly had the much healthier relationship to the sport. She competed to do *her* best. She didn't need to become *the* best. She wasn't obsessed with taking it to the next level. It wasn't only about winning (or not losing) to her.

When I think of Carly's approach, "self-preservation" is the word that comes to mind. Skating was never more important to her than her own well-being. What separated us was something that the Olympic champion Scott Hamilton described as the invisible step: the elevation of one's motivation from improving to winning, which elevates an athlete's intensity from a 10 on a 1-to-10 scale to a 15. Carly maintained boundaries that I lacked. She didn't see the point of throwing herself into the air fifty or sixty times in a single session to land a single jump perfectly. She was not motivated to commit to an off-ice program of strength training *and* spin classes *and* hot yoga sessions *and* ballet four or five times a week so that she could see a fractional improvement on the ice.

She was content to chase personal milestones. She did not need national titles or Olympic berths to justify her existence. She could finish fifth and if she had put forth her best effort, she was happy. I was mystified by her healthy attitude and ability to self-regulate because I had neither. I *needed* the medals and titles in some way, to validate that I really was good and that the effort was worth it. Her internal compass is not the norm in a sport like skating, where the most obvious measures of success are dependent on the opinions of other people—namely, the judges.

If I did my best and finished fifth, it would be the worst outcome imaginable. If my best effort is good enough for only fifth, what am I doing here? If I'm not capable of winning, what's the point? That's where I was coming from. It was a mindset encouraged by my parents, who always counseled us that anything worth doing was worth doing really, really well.

Their desire to see us succeed was genuine but not entirely selfless. Our victories became a validation of their parenting, which I picked up on years later after I made the Olympic team and my dad was interviewed for a feature that ran in his hometown newspaper, *The Joplin Globe*. The headline: "Former Joplin Man's Daughter to Go for Skating Gold in Sochi."

A psychologist I saw in my teens once gave my mom a homework assignment: read the 2001 book *The Blessing of a Skinned Knee* by Wendy Mogel, a child psychologist. As I understand it, the book encourages parents to see past their children's talents and appreciate all the ways in which they are ordinary, the better to relate to them as perfectly imperfect human beings.

I don't remember Mom ever completing that assignment.

Some people study their parents to make sense of their physical traits—their curly hair or beaked nose. I look at Denise and Carl Gold for clues to understand where my behaviors come from.

My parents met at the hospital in Missouri where they both worked. If I close my eyes, I can picture their meet-cute moment: the petite and vivacious nurse catching the eye of the socially awkward doctor. They fell in love while married to other people (an inconvenient fact that would come back to haunt Mom). My mom is a California-born flower child, and my dad is a conservative midwesterner, so it's a mystery to me how they ended up together. I know now that alcohol lubricated their connection.

As a child I remember straight-out asking them both what attracted each to the other and being perplexed when they sidestepped my question. My best guess as an adult—since they still won't talk about it—is they were the hot party couple that ran with the fast crowd and bonded over last calls.

I can't blame my mom for seeing my dad as a promising project, a secondhand partner that she could rehabilitate like all her thrift-store treasures. She came of age at a time when women did not have the freedoms or choices that Carly and I take for granted. She couldn't obtain her first credit card unless her husband or father co-signed the application. The careers available to women outside the house were pretty limited. Her best chance at upward mobility wasn't a job, it was a marriage to an upwardly mobile man, and cultural forces conditioned her to believe that putting her most attractive foot forward required being the thinnest version of herself. Mom was taught, as women still are, that smallness equaled strength.

I've never known Mom to go a single day giving herself permission to eat whatever she desires. Cheat days are foreign to her. She is the mom who pops two or three almonds into her mouth and calls it lunch; who considers half a grapefruit and coffee a complete meal; who insists that fresh fruit is as sweet as any sugary dessert; who takes two bites of turkey and one bite of mashed potatoes at Thanksgiving before pushing her plate away and groaning, "I'm stuffed."

Her discipline has paid off. She's sixty-nine as I write this and could easily pass for someone in her forties. My father couldn't resist her, and he ticked off a lot of her boxes, too. He had been a star athlete in high school in football, basketball, and track before pursuing a career in medicine. As a doctor, he figured to provide Mom with the financial security she wanted not just for herself but for her children. She had grown up piss-poor and was determined to give us a better start. And he was great with Kendra, Mom's daughter from her first marriage, who was born nearly twenty years before me and Carly. Theirs was, at least on paper, a fairy-tale marriage, which made it tricky when life got real.

The narrative of our existence, fed to us in loving spoonfuls by Mom, was that we were her miracle babies. She had prayed so hard for us, had wanted us desperately, and as such was happy to stay at home and make our care her full-time occupation. From the outside, it looked like Carly and I lacked for nothing. We had a menagerie of pets, which at one point included dogs, cats, a hedgehog, and a chinchilla—and our parents' full attention. Any activity that we expressed an interest in, Mom and Dad threw their whole support behind it.

Like most children, Carly and I weren't privy to aspects of our parents' lives and marriage that might have helped us make sense of how they related to each other. Knowing what I know now, I can see how Mom became more emotionally attached to me and Carly as she became more disconnected from Dad. We were clueless as kids because our parents did their best to keep the ugly stuff from us to give us the carefree childhoods that they hadn't had.

And we did have some wonderful times. One of my absolute favorite memories is of a family trip we took to Cancún. It was right before I started skating, so I'm going to say that Carly and I were seven. We stayed at a fancy resort and swam with dolphins. We got our hair braided and burned ourselves to a crisp at the beach during the day and played Pictionary at night. Mom and Dad refrained from yelling, for the most part. Everyone was *happy.*

It was the last vacation I can remember us taking that wasn't skating-related. Later, I would connect skating with the unraveling of our family, which was like blaming a tornado for the destruction of a shoddily built house. My family's foundation was crumbling at least as far back as our preschool years when Mom found out Dad was cheating on her after the damning evidence arrived in the mail, wedged between the weekly circulars and bills. A hotel nearby had kindly returned my father's driver's license, which he had forgotten to collect at the front desk.

The biggest piece of the puzzle, the one hidden from me and Carly for a long time, was that Dad had had a substance abuse problem that was serious enough to land him in a treatment center before we were born. And that Mom had been a drinker, too. Our parents moved past their party days, but I'm not sure they ever processed whatever traumas drove them to all those bars and all that booze. Neither was great at managing their emotions in a healthy way, and the added stresses of parenthood mixed with their own discordant personalities turned them into walking powder kegs.

Especially Dad. On the one hand, he was our Tickle Monster and co-conspirator in junk food raids. I used to think that he set out to be the "fun" parent as a means to win our love, but as I've gotten older it's occurred to me that he let us stay up late and eat pizza—even at competitions, when how we fuel our bodies became doubly important—because *he* wanted to stay up late. *He* wanted to eat pizza and junk food. It was about satisfying his desires instead of considering what's best for us.

I've *never* eaten a Butterfinger candy bar in front of my mom, and even now, I shudder to think how she'd react if she found an empty chocolate wrapper under my bed. But at least she was/is coming from a place of what's best for us nutrition-wise. Dad, on the other hand, would let me order a pizza at ten at night, drink a liter of regular soda before bed, and stay up way, way, way past my bedtime to sit on the couch with him and watch horror movies that would spark nightmares once I finally did go to sleep.

I remember watching *Bram Stoker's Dracula* when I was four years old. It wasn't rated R for restful, that's for sure. Nothing like a gothic horror film to send me off to sleep. I imagined green mist creeping into my bedroom for weeks afterward. Around this time, my night terrors began. I'd wake up in tears but not in my bed. *Where am I? How did I get here?* I had no idea. I was a fidgety, foot-tapping bundle of anxiety. I bit my nails until my cuticles bled. I had my extreme sensory issues. I'd routinely erupt into kicking, screaming, punching rages that would prompt Mom or Dad to drop everything and come running to comfort me.

But here's the thing. Dad could be scarier than Gary Oldman's Dracula. He had a hair-trigger temper that terrified me. I remember one weekend outing with Dad when Carly and I were eleven or twelve. We had finished dinner and he was driving us to the movies. I was in the front seat, riding shotgun, which was my normal spot. Carly was in her usual seat directly behind Dad. One minute I was being sassy, running my mouth and pushing Dad's buttons. Next thing I knew, he had tightened his grip on the wheel with his left hand, grabbed my left shoulder with his right hand, and was shaking me. He shoved me into the passenger-side window as he screamed, with eyes as dark as coal, "Look at me when I'm talking to you!" I fell silent. Not another word was uttered until we were inside the movie theater. Then it was as if nothing had ever happened. "You girls want popcorn? A soda?"

Mom's swings of emotions could be just as intense. In her fifties, she experienced a pain radiating out from her hip that was so excruciating, she believed that she might have bone cancer. She never said anything about it to us, so when she was impatient with us or flew off the handle, Carly and I blamed ourselves. We bent over backward to placate her, believing we were the cause of her misery. Imagine Mom's relief when her cascading physical issues were ascribed to an arthritic left hip, bad but fixable with replacement surgery. But when she told us about the procedure, I remember Carly and I were both shocked. How could Mom be in so much pain without us knowing?

I think about those days a lot, and what stands out is the underlying melancholy that permeated our family's existence. But because no allowances were made for unhappiness in our household—we were steeped in the fake-it-till-you-make-it culture—that sadness got expressed as anger.

More than once, I can remember us driving to a competition, and Mom and Dad would be screaming at each other. Carly and I'd ask, "What's wrong?" and Mom would blurt out, "Ask your father!" These exchanges followed the same pattern: harsh words leading to verbal explosions followed by long silences, sullen faces, and sometimes tears.

And then we'd pull into the parking lot, put on big smiles, open our doors, and walk into the rink.

My ability to project to the world a flawless image was a critical component of my skating success, and I can thank my parents for modeling how to put on a public face that projects calm and poise no matter what kind of shit's going down behind the scenes. The importance in skating of putting your best foot forward and of staying in that character cannot be overestimated. You are being judged on and off the ice. It's a *performance* in the strictest sense of the word. You learn to monitor your behavior at all times because the judges' eyes are always on you. They register what you wear, what you eat in the hotel restaurant, how you act in public. And while you're the main character, everyone in your family has a part to play. If any dysfunction is on display, it can negatively affect how you are judged on the ice, because the people who decide our competitive fates are looking for the complete package in their champions.

I internalized from my parents that to be liked or accepted, I should keep my ugly parts hidden. All those big feelings I had weren't going to win me any friends or influence people. Best to keep them stuffed down. A funny thing about that: I could deny my own feelings, but I was hyperaware of those of everyone around me. I was a goddamn human thermometer, always calibrating the temperature in the room. But it sometimes led to faulty readings. One time when I was still in juniors, I returned to the hotel room after an awful performance and walked in to find my father sobbing. He gave no reason for why he was so upset. Looking back, I think it probably involved some secret he had been keeping from Mom that had come to light. But I didn't know any better then. I assumed he was reacting to my bad result. *I was such a loser I made my father cry!*

When things were bad between them, Mom would shut down. She'd be there but not be there. Physically present but emotionally somewhere else. We'd ask her over and over what was wrong. "Nothing," she said. "Don't worry," she said. "Just focus on your skating." But it was obvious something was not right.

One time, I remember, Carly decided to snoop around and get to the bottom of things. When Mom was in another room, Carly grabbed her phone, scrolled through it, and stumbled upon an exchange with Dad in which Mom accused him of cheating on her. When Carly confronted Mom about it, she confirmed: "Your father is having affairs. He's an asshole. There. Are you happy now?"

We were devastated. To discover that Dad wasn't who we thought he was, to learn that he was stepping out on Mom, was a lot to process. I was pulled in different directions by the revelation. I was sad but also angry at both of them. To Mom, I wanted to say, *I know you just found out that Dad cheated on you again, but why is that our fault? Why are you taking it out on us?*

And Dad, well, he was a fucking cliché, cheating on Mom, mostly with people he met at work who were basically younger versions of her (one woman was even named Denise).

As my public profile grew, his affairs were doubly mortifying. Carly and I saw texts on his phone where he was talking about my competitions with his mistress of the month or—grosser still—live-texting with her from one of my events. From what we read, it seemed pretty clear that he was trading off being my dad to impress someone he wanted to bed. It made me sick to my stomach to consider that somewhere a woman might be watching me skate on TV and saying, *That's the daughter of the man I'm fucking.*

What made this so, so much worse was that on paper, the Golds looked good. Midwestern strong. United. We knew our roles, and for a long time we played them to perfection.

"I work in a hospital," my dad told the *New York Post* in 2014, "and I deal with life and death and I've got the easy job." Mom, he said, "is the engine that drives the train and keeps it on the track." That was the setup. Dad was the Provider. Mom was the Protector. Carly was the Peacemaker. And me? I was the Golds' gift to the world. Don't believe me? Dad spelled it out in a birthday letter he wrote to me on my twenty-third birthday: "You came to us, and the rest of the world, as an unmerited gift from God Almighty himself!"

Yeah, but was I the gift? Or was my skating the gift? If my parents' love for me and Carly was unconditional, why were they infinitely more invested in my results than Carly's? It bothered me that she never felt equally supported. It's one of my biggest sorrows, because she was talented in her own right. You can look it up. In 2016, she was crowned the Pacific Coast Sectional senior ladies' champion. It's a prestigious title that had been won the previous year by the future national champion and Olympian Karen Chen (past winners included Peggy Fleming and Michelle Kwan). If Carly's surname had been Smith, she would have merited national attention. Instead, she often felt invisible—including in her own family. So many of her competitions she attended by herself because Mom was off somewhere with me and Dad was unreliable. She'd be in the locker room after competing, so excited to tell us how she'd done, and no one would pick up their phone. Even when we were there to support Carly, we often came up short. I remember one time Mom and I slept through Carly's short program at her regionals because we were jet-lagged.

We weren't the first sporting family to mask family dysfunction with flight. But every move we made had downstream effects, carrying me farther from my non-skating friends, academia, normalcy. The stakes for me grew exponentially with every sacrifice made by everybody else to advance my career. The pressure I felt to succeed to validate the decisions made by my parents on my behalf became intense. I was a teenage girl in a body-conscious sport untethered from a traditional school and home. What could go wrong?

I recognize that my relentless drive and determination put my mom and dad in a tough spot. What loving parent wouldn't endeavor to do everything humanly possible to help make their child's dreams come true? Maybe my parents could have pumped the brakes and avoided tearing apart our family—or at least recognized when the people and culture were toxic and taking their toll on me. But it's tricky. Because there's no guarantee that I wouldn't have ended up resenting like hell that they had held me back. Sadly, I ended up resenting them anyway.

3

SHORT TEMPERS AND BIG HEARTS

At fourteen years old, I arrived at a fork in the road. As a novice, I had just finished fourth at the 2010 U.S. Championships in Spokane, Washington, which had earned me a medal. It was a big deal. The boys' novice winner that year was future Olympic champion Nathan Chen. Most, if not all, of the other girls in the top ten were being homeschooled, so their days could revolve around skating. My parents, once vehemently opposed to the idea of taking Carly and me out of regular school, capitulated. If I wanted to see how far skating could carry me, skating, not school, had to provide the ballast of my days.

Starting in our sophomore year, Carly and I attended our classes online. And my skating got . . . worse. I took a step backward when I finished sixth at the midwestern sectionals during the 2010–11 season and failed to qualify for nationals again. I barely completed a clean jumping pass and fell four times in my free skate. At fifteen years old I was having to confront the possibility that juniors was the end of the line for me in skating. In every athletic career there are these moments of reckoning.

Maybe you exceed the limits of what your body can endure. Or your priorities or circumstances shift. Or you simply fall out of love with your sport. Though it's all part of the natural order of things, it was traumatic for my whole family since our daily lives had become so entwined with my skating

To paraphrase Simon Joyner paraphrasing Flannery O'Connor, I had arrived at the point where people are forced to make a decision that either enables them to transcend a circumstance or leads them to succumb to it. I was shocked and confused. I believed in my heart that I could be a top-level skater, but my poor finish forced me to confront the possibility that my optimism outstripped my abilities. Carly took it harder than I did. She was *sobbing.* Mom was also beside herself. I think it was because our emotional circuitry was so intertwined. It was as if my devastation was their own.

What felt like the end of the world was, in fact, the start of puberty. I experienced a six-inch growth spurt in a matter of months that vaulted me to five foot four. My knees ached. My hip flexors felt like taut rubber bands ready to snap. It felt like I was inhabiting a new body, and it took a while for me to adjust to my new center of gravity. I lost confidence as I gained height.

Mom would describe the days that followed as a "little bit of a grieving process." It was quite possible that what we were mourning wasn't just a lost season but a fading dream. Skating is hard to begin with, and when you tack on the normal stresses related to the intense biological changes ushered in by puberty, it creates a logical stopping point for most girls, especially those already susceptible to the allure of a so-called normal teenage life.

My mom gave me an out. She told me she only wanted me to be happy. She reassured me that I didn't have to be a figure skater. "For all the time and money we're putting into your skating, you could be great at something else," she said.

She was assuming that I equated happiness with greatness. I don't know. At that stage in my life, that was probably true. Of course, I sometimes wished I could gather with friends after school and waste away the afternoon gorging on gossip and meat-lovers' deep-dish pizzas. On occasion I wanted to stay up late bingeing *American Horror Story* instead of making sure I got the nine hours of sleep my body needed to function well on the ice. But ultimately, I still really liked skating. And there was also the small matter that Carly and I had no regular school to fall back on. My school friends and I weren't as close now that I wasn't attending classes in person. My entire world essentially revolved around the rink. My parents' worlds, too. What would our lives look like without skating? What would we bond over? I had come this far. What was it that Yoda told Luke in *The Empire Strikes Back*? "Do. Or do not. There is no try." I didn't want to quit on skating just yet.

As Mom would say, it was a nervy situation.

To ease my path moving forward, Mom researched sports psychologists and found one for me to talk to. Her name was Jenny and she was a gem. She worked with me to view my performances through a softer lens: It can be lonely on the ice. You're out there by yourself, just you and your music and all the results you're terrified of. She helped me to temper my darkest thoughts. She's very special to me because she didn't just save me. She was a godsend to Carly, validating her experience by helping her to see with clear eyes her role in the family as the invisible child, the dark matter that held us together. Jenny saved Carly, who in turn would save me from myself time and again.

And in the end, Jenny would swoop in to save me from the man who in 2011 encouraged me to get up off the canvas and keep fighting. His name was Alex Ouriashev, and I had begun working with him in my early teens. He came recommended by another coach I worked with at Cruella's rink. I have nothing but fond memories of this woman, who was kind and compassionate and restored my faith in skating, broadly, and in coaches, specifically, after I escaped Cruella's clutches. She was a very important caregiver to me in my transition from Cruella to Alex. She was probably the most holistic of all the coaches I had, but after I landed a clean triple Lutz on my third attempt, she pushed me to work with Alex, having recognized that she couldn't take me any further in the sport. And so, with Mom behind the wheel, I began making the 200-mile drive from Springfield to Chicagoland, where Alex was based, to be coached by him on a part-time basis. We started out working together a few times a month and kept adding sessions until Carly, Mom, and I were basically living out of a suitcase at a hotel near his rink.

Alex was a native of Ukraine and by the time we started working together, he was nearing sixty and was a naturalized citizen of the United States, where he had lived for more than twenty-five years. He could see that he had a challenge on his hands. I had great lift on my jumps, thanks to my natural athletic ability, but once I was airborne my arms were all over the place, calling to mind the waving inflatable tube men you see at car dealership lots. Alex wasn't quite sure where to start with refining my technique, but he was charmed by my personality and enthusiasm and decided I was well worth his time and effort.

I definitely considered him one of the best jumping technicians in the country, if not the world, and if others didn't see him that way, it's probably because he didn't seek the spotlight. Which might have been for the best given what happened when it found him.

In the beginning, I felt fortunate to be able to drink from the well of his knowledge. Growing up in the old Soviet system, Alex had been schooled in technique by masters. He was a stickler for details. He kept a notebook in which he documented the particulars of every jump I attempted in practice, recording the altitude, the precision of the entrance, and the exactness of the landing.

Alas, Alex also kept a record of our weights and heights, the latter of which I always thought was odd since we couldn't will ourselves to be taller or shorter. The summer of my growth spurt, the number on the scale seemed to jump overnight. Alex would make the occasional comment about how my butt looked big, which irritated my mother—until she glanced around the rink and noticed that all the other skaters *were* pretty thin. Around this time, Mom started weighing Carly and me at home, which makes her look like a shitty parent. It wasn't her finest hour, but in her defense, she was weighing herself all the time, too. Many ugly wars were waged on the battleground that was our bathroom scale, and I learned the hard way that shaming works. There was nothing like a high number to trigger behavior modifications.

Alex had been a two-time senior men's national champion in his home country. He had had the talent to make the USSR Olympic team back in the day, he told me, but he hadn't worked hard enough to make it happen. And now it was too late. He'd live the rest of his life with his regrets. He didn't want that ending for me. "Trust process," he said.

I had faith in Alex. So instead of quitting after that disastrous sectionals, I doubled down. Mom, Carly, and I found an apartment to rent near the rinks that Alex used for teaching, and once again we left Dad behind. I hadn't realized how much the vagabond life had been wearing on me until I was sprung from it.

Once we were settled in our suburban Chicago apartment, my training became more consistent. I was getting more and better rest and adjusting to my new center of gravity. The jumps came back, stronger than ever, and I strung together some excellent performances early in the 2011–12 season. I made my international debut at a Junior Grand Prix event in Estonia and won, returned to the sectionals where I had flamed out the year prior and won that, too, and then added the junior title at nationals with the highest score that had ever been recorded in the competition's junior ladies' division.

Mitch Moyer was U.S. Figure Skating's senior director of athlete high performance at the time, and he had been tracking my progress since he first saw me compete at the novice level at nationals. By the time I won the junior title and followed it with a silver-medal performance at the World Junior Championships in Minsk, Belarus, he was excited about my potential. In his mind, I had everything: the jumps, the looks, the name. All I lacked was international experience—well, that and eye makeup. My lack of eye shadow and mascara seemed a much bigger deal than even the thinness of my senior-level resume. It was certainly remarked upon a lot more often.

Mitch would rectify my lack of experience with a move that raised some eyebrows. When a spot unexpectedly opened up in a prestigious competition called the World Team Trophy, he sent me to Tokyo in April 2012 to participate. It was like promoting a Triple-A baseball player to the majors for a playoff game. I finished fifth and—red flag alert—was devastated because I had skated a poor free skate and believed I had let down my older teammates.

Around this time I also landed on the radar of the International Management Group, which added me to its stable of athletes when I was sixteen. IMG's interest stamped me as a prospective star. It telegraphed to everyone in skating that I was someone worth investing in. In one year's time, I had gone from the verge of quitting to the cusp of stardom. Life was coming at me fast.

In 2013, I advanced to my first nationals in senior ladies' singles. The competition was in Omaha, Nebraska. I skated a horrible short program to place ninth. When I met up with my mom and Carly in the CenturyLink Center concourse, they did their best to put a positive spin on things, but I was inconsolable. I dug my very expensive skates out of my bag and chucked them against the wall.

Now, it's one thing if you're the tennis player Nick Kyrgios and you break a couple of rackets on the court after a tough loss at the U.S. Open. But imagine if he had carried his rackets up to the concourse level of Arthur Ashe Stadium and *then* slammed them to the ground. I was lucky I didn't hit anybody and that nobody was around to videotape my behavior and turn me into an unflattering meme on social media. It was also a miracle both blades survived the impact.

Having released all that pent-up frustration, I went out and won the free skate to finish second to my future rival Ashley Wagner to establish myself as a legitimate contender for a 2014 Olympics berth. The pattern by then was long-established: Fiasco. Implosion. Redemption. Equanimity. As I like to say, I was always playing with F.I.R.E. Anger is a powerful emotion, and it gave me strength, energy, and power, at least in the short term. The problem with using anger as fuel is it's not sustainable. Eventually, the anger will cannibalize your performance—and, possibly, your sanity.

In the spring and summer of 2013, I worked harder than I ever had. I'd remain on the ice after everyone else was done, ignoring the Zamboni driver waiting to resurface the ice because I needed to repeat my triple Lutz–triple toe combination until it was just right. Mom would sit near the ice dutifully recording each combination on my phone so I could review it afterward. One time, I scrolled through all the jumps and counted fifty-five failed attempts followed by one that was perfect. The fifty-sixth time was a charm.

Alex recognized the compulsions that made me tick because he shared them. It's wild, if you think about it: a man plucked from his home as a child to be developed into a champion sportsman in the old state-sponsored Soviet system finding a kindred spirit in the American girl raised in freedom who gladly sacrificed her childhood to do the same. Perhaps because of this connection, he molded me into a jumper whom people compared to Tonya Harding. Anyone who saw her become the first American woman to land a triple Axel in competition knew what a huge compliment that was.

Alex's coaching methods were admittedly unconventional. In one of my favorite drills, he'd pit me against the best male skater at the club and engage us in timed jumping games. I remember winning one contest by executing seventeen double Axels in thirty seconds (if you singled or underrotated a jump, it didn't count). Another time, I prevailed by executing all six triples (Axel, Salchow, toe loop, loop, flip, and Lutz) in twenty-four seconds. Alex loved this game. I did, too. It was an inventive way to build endurance and speed while sharpening our competitiveness. I liked that you could quantitatively track your improvement from week to week.

Alex also expressed genuine interest in my life away from the rink. He'd ask me what music I was listening to, what clothing I liked, what movies I had seen. It was a big deal, all that small talk. Maybe it's partly a consequence of ice time being so precious, but my experience with skating coaches is that they are generally all business. They interact with their skaters as if the skaters are au-

more times than not, whoever ended up with the short straw burst into tears.

I'd run through my programs, nonstop (theoretically) from start to finish, and I was not allowed more than a single mistake. If I made two or more, he would order every skater on the session—not just me—to run laps around the building as punishment. His two-mistakes-for-Gracie, running-for-all approach was his way of simulating the stress of competing. It was the old Soviet way. No pressure like peer pressure. Whatever his reasoning, it was not exactly conducive to team bonding. When the other skaters shot me dirty looks as we huffed and puffed around the building, I wanted to scream, *Believe it or not, it was not my goal to fuck up on all my jumps today to make you run!*

Did I mention that if everybody else had to run ten laps, I'd be made to do twenty? Whenever I complained, Alex would explain that I couldn't expect to achieve special things if I did the same thing as everybody else. Sometimes he would follow me in his car while I ran to make sure I didn't take any shortcuts.

Our off-ice core sessions were another sore spot. We'd be executing crunches or holding a boat pose and Alex would step on our stomachs. This was his idea of toughening us up because that's how he had been trained. Alex was forever reminding us that we were getting off easy. He'd share stories from his training in Moscow. In addition to the rink, the facility had a swimming pool that the figure skating coaches incorporated into their conditioning program. Alex and his fellow skaters would put on their swimsuits and hop into the deep water, expel all the air in their lungs, and descend to the bottom, where they'd remain, arms linked so nobody could drift off if they fainted, for ninety seconds at a time. It was Soviet Union water torture disguised as a hypoxic breathing exercise intended to boost the body's red blood cell count and improve endurance. As one of the younger skaters, Alex said he lived in constant fear that he would faint and cause them all to have to repeat the drill.

I remember saying, "Alex, what's the moral of this story?" I loved skating, but not enough to risk passing out in the deep end of a pool just to improve my lung capacity for the final minute of my free skate. There's stamina and then there's insanity. It was hard to say back then where I'd draw the line at doing whatever was necessary to improve, but that, I decided, might be it.

I'm sure there were parents who questioned Alex's "mad genius" and its expression in his authoritarian methods. My mom was sometimes one of them. She wasn't the type to stand along the sideboards and yell out instructions like some other parents. She left the coaching to Alex unless she believed he had overstepped a boundary. For example, Alex added a thirty-minute run to my weekend schedule, and he'd phone my mom to check up on me and make sure that I completed it. Mom always told him I did, even when she knew I hadn't. I didn't want to put her in the position of having to lie, so most weeks I'd drive out to the nearest track and spend thirty minutes listening to music, then return home. That way, when Mom asked where I had been, I could say, truthfully, "I was at the track." I whiled away hundreds of hours as a teenager hiding in my car behind a building adjacent to the running oval.

But there were other times when Mom would cut me no slack. She'd harshly question my motivation if I popped several jumps in a session or looked sluggish. If that makes her sound like the worst type of tiger mom, all I can say is a certain amount of pushing is necessary to mold a great athlete into an Olympian, and in the process it's easy for a supportive parent to morph into a meddler. This is especially true when you're in a culture, as exists in elite sports, where unquestioned devotion is demanded, creating an untenable dissonance when you have internal doubts about actions that everyone else accepts in good faith. The badgering is considered a kind of love language. I remember one of my coaches in Springfield, Missouri, when I was just starting out, pushing me to repeat drills until I was exhausted. At eight years old, I was absorbing the lesson that I couldn't just sit on the ice and cry. If I wanted to be an Olympian, I had to pick myself up and do a drill over and over and over.

From the start, it was instilled in me that if you want to be better than everybody else, you can't allow yourself to be comfortable, not for a single day. In this environment, the line between motivational tactics and abuse can be as thin as a skating blade. It's easy to cross without realizing it.

I often pictured Alex, not my father, walking me down the aisle at my wedding. That's how much he meant to me. I considered him family. But that was before every day became all or nothing. If I skated well, he lavished me with praise. "The best in the world," he'd call me. The next day, I'd struggle and the bouquets would be replaced by withering critiques. "Look at your butt," he'd say. "You're too heavy."

Really? How could I go from best in the world to too fat to fly in twenty-four hours? It was absurd. In the spring of 2013, I returned from Japan, where I had toured with an ice show for a month. I practiced between performances, but those sessions were not nearly as intense as my usual routine. And we were eating a lot of meals on the go, so it wasn't too shocking that when I finally got home and stepped on the scale, I had put on five pounds.

I resumed my workouts with Alex, which meant the return of the daily weigh-in. That first day, the needle stopped north of 125 pounds. Alex, then as big and soft as a hibernating bear, looked up and said gravely, "That's big number, Gracie."

I was five foot four, remember, most of it muscle, which would put me at the low end of normal on the BMI. As I resumed intense training, the extra pounds probably would have melted off me. Alex could have monitored my weight without making a big deal of it. He knows now that he handled it all wrong.

I didn't mind Alex's directness when he said, "You're taller than you used to be and that's why you're struggling with this jump." If I fell on a triple flip, what was Alex supposed to do, applaud my effort? For all its elegance, skating is a rough-and-tumble sport. If you mistake anything other than flattery as cruelty, don't bother skating. That's always been my mindset, which is probably why I worked so well with Alex for so long.

But when he said, "You're heavier than you used to be and that's why you're struggling with this jump," it triggered me. My height I couldn't control. It was predetermined by genetics, so I didn't feel defensive about it. But my weight? I was brought up to see that as something I should be able to control through sheer willpower. Hadn't I spent years watching Mom maintain her girlish figure through self-discipline and rigid dieting? So when Alex commented on my *shape*, I felt shame. My mom's vigilance over her figure had signaled to me that being unable to control one's weight wasn't about nutrition or biology. It was a goddamn character flaw.

There was so much chaos baked into the Alex experience. On occasion, he would miss practice. Just fail to show up. At least once, I can remember Mom driving to his apartment and banging on his door to try unsuccessfully to summon him. Other times he'd show up reeking of what I thought was a cologne, a sort of sweet, sort of spicy scent that I could never place because of its distinctiveness—until the first time I opened a bottle of cognac, long after we had stopped working together. And then the recognition hit me like a triple shot of espresso. *This is what Alex smelled like.*

The cologne that I could never positively identify was alcohol.

Alex is open about his drinking now. He describes it as a bad, stupid thing that everyone in his generation did where he grew up. He has since sworn off alcohol, but when we were working together his drinking was a problem. He became someone I barely recognized. One day he launched into a familiar tirade at the end of a mistake-filled practice: "How are you going to beat the Russians with those jumps? You don't have really good jumps like theirs. How are you going to beat Yuna Kim with those spins? Hers are beautiful."

He meant it as a motivational message, but he had read me all wrong. To be compared unfavorably to my main competitors by the one person I wanted to please more than anybody else in the world was thoroughly deflating.

He also used to say, "If you skate like that, you shouldn't wear a Team USA jacket. This skating is for Team Mexico." It was cruel and condescending and racist. The bully trifecta.

The final straw was Cannoli-gate. Carly and I turned eighteen in August, and Mom brought to the rink a fancy bakery-bought cake consisting of a giant cannoli packed with miniature cannoli that could be easily extracted. It was a nice gesture because our birthdays tended to go off the rails.

Our seventeenth birthday was a case in point. Dad had made plans to join us for what was by then a rare family meal. At skating that day, I couldn't do anything right. Not so Carly, who flew across the ice. Her legs were like springs, her jumps were textbook perfect. She was pumped. I was in tears afterward, and Mom was furious. She harangued me all the way home about my lack of focus while Carly stewed in the backseat. Once again, her achievements were second to mine, never important enough to deflect or defuse the complete meltdowns from me or Mom. Nobody cared that she had had a great practice. All that mattered was that I was a hot mess. My struggles, not her satisfaction, ruled the day.

Upon arriving home, Carly lost it. "What about me?" she said. She was sobbing. "Does what I do not matter?" It pained me to see Carly so upset. I stormed upstairs, screaming at Mom for driving Carly to tears, completely ignoring Dad, who was on the couch, as useless as a decorative pillow. I failed to realize that Mom was close on my heels. Too close, evidently, because when I stormed into my bedroom and slammed the door, I gave Mom a corneal abrasion. Sobbing, she called me a monster. Dad sat there saying nothing. I slipped out of the house and walked around the block to remove myself from the explosion that I'd just caused, muttering the whole way that literally everything wrong with my family was my fault.

And Carly? She was frantically scrolling through restaurant websites online, looking for somewhere—anywhere—that would accept a last-minute reservation for four because our original slot had come and gone. She found a restaurant and we drove there in total silence, ate in total silence, returned home in total silence. Mom stomped upstairs to sulk. Dad sat back down on the coach and stared at his phone, staying out of the fight because, as he said, he "always made it worse," but really because he was so uninvolved in our lives by this point he'd rather check out and text his mistress of the month.

Carly was devastated that her birthday got ruined yet again and that—surprise!—our parents clearly didn't see her. And I was absolutely livid that my skating had the power to make or break everything, and that my mom was painting herself as the victim and me as the problem.

But when we all woke up the next day, we pretended—in pure Gold fashion—as if nothing had happened.

Now it was a year later and Mom had bought this gorgeous cannoli cake. It was so thoughtful of her. I was genuinely excited. Maybe this year was going to be different. This birthday and my next year on the planet were going to be epic.

And then Alex had to go and ruin everything.

All the other skaters had exited the ice and gathered in the party room for the cutting of the cannoli cake and the opening of presents. I moved to step off the ice, and Alex stopped me. I could have my cake *after* the Olympics, he said. But right now I had more training to do.

He made me stay on the ice even after I had powered through my short program run-through, even after I had powered through all my jumps. I burst into tears because I was so fucking tired and as usual I could never do enough to please Alex. The thought of peering through the plexiglass as everyone sang "Happy Birthday" to Carly and watched her open gifts was the final indignity. He had broken me.

Mom was pissed. She explained to Alex that she had made reservations for us to go zip-lining and we had to leave by the bottom of the hour, and the longer he kept me on the ice, the less time I was going to have for cake. I'm sure it was only because of her intercession that I was allowed to get off the ice and join the party. I reached for a slice of the fancy cake, and Alex slapped my hand in front of everybody. "Do you really think you should be having cake?" he asked. Mom heard him and muttered under her breath, "It's her birthday. Just let her have some cake."

The day pretty much went downhill from there. We made it to zip-lining, but only because Dad took the wheel and raced like a Formula One driver, swerving around other cars and weaving through lanes while Mom screamed at him to be careful and

Carly and I cowered in fright. We arrived at our destination with tearstained cheeks; Mom's face was frozen in a scowl, and Dad was genuinely clueless as to why no one was congratulating him on making record time.

Zip-lining wasn't the scariest thing I did that day. Parting ways with Alex was.

I was on the verge of making the Olympics—and of burning out. If this daily abuse was the price I had to pay for becoming an Olympian, I decided then maybe I wasn't cut out to be one. I told Mom that I'd rather quit the sport than continue training with Alex.

Mom had an intense conversation with Jenny, the psychologist, who backed me up. She expressed in no uncertain terms that it was a good move—a necessary one, even—for me to seek a new coach if I was going to continue in the sport. Hers was not a view widely shared by those inside U.S. Figure Skating. I arrived at the annual conditioning camp in Colorado Springs, Colorado, the next day without Alex, who stayed home after I told him that we were through. The way officials reacted, you would have thought I came without my skates and not my ex-coach.

The officials were shocked that I showed up with my mom by my side but no Alex. They were concerned that I had no plan for who would coach me next. They seemed unmoved by my explanation that Alex's verbal and emotional abuse had gone too far. They wondered why I couldn't "just make it work" until after the Olympics. Nobody seemed to notice that I was heartbroken. Marina Zoueva and Oleg Epstein, two Detroit-based coaches, accompanied me to the ice so I wouldn't be alone.

It is almost unheard of to switch coaches and cities so close to the Olympics. If anything, skaters are inclined to lean even deeper into routine. I remember officials interceding to try to patch things up between me and Alex. I stood my ground. My mom and I flew home, packed up our apartment, and left.

If not for Alex, I never would have become an Olympian. He was the Dr. Frankenstein behind the creation of Gracie Gold. That's a fact. But if I had stayed with him, I never would have made it to Sochi. In the quest to mold me into the best version of myself, he nearly destroyed me.

The last year of our collaboration was the dawning of my realization that to be a great artist, a great athlete, it helps to embrace behaviors that are neither ordinary nor particularly healthy. You are, after all, attempting to achieve something that, if you think about it, is a little insane. Have you heard the story of Vincent van Gogh and the yellow paint? I read somewhere that van Gogh, a depressive, drank yellow paint because he thought if his insides were coated with the color that calls to mind warmth and sunshine, he'd feel better. I look back at my final months with Alex as my van Gogh period. Triple Lutzes were my yellow paint. If I did ten in a row, I'd feel good. If I did twenty or thirty, I'd feel better. Each triple chemically rewarded my adolescent brain like a double dose of dopamine.

Neither van Gogh with his lead-based paint nor I with my lighter-is-tighter jumps had the clarity of thought to recognize that the very act we thought was improving our well-being was actually making us more unwell. But in the short term, the dieting, the perfectionism, and the enthusiastic embrace of the role of Gracie Gold that coalesced in Chicagoland were about to pay off big-time.

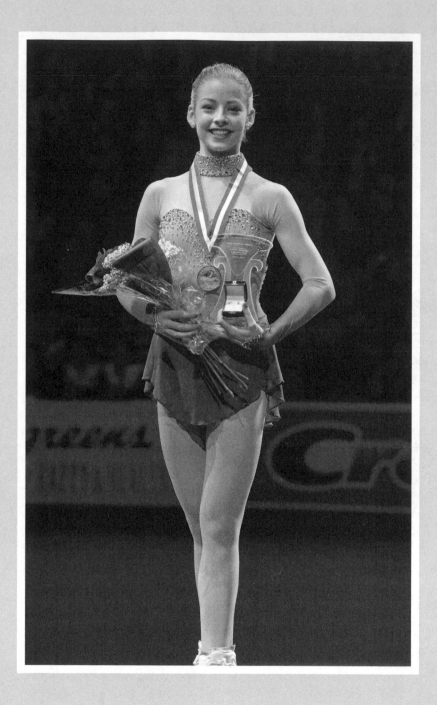

GRACIE GOLD

PART TWO

Then he said: Don't you know? I am trying to
make you great.
And I said: I do not want to be great, I want
to be loved.

—SUE ZHAO

4

"DO YOUR JOB"

"She's a gorgeous girl. She looks like Grace Kelly."

With that assessment, offered ahead of the 2014 Olympics, my coach Frank Carroll unveiled a new monster: Gracie Gold.

Frank insists that the comparison had been in the ether. All he did was bottle it up and serve it to reporters, but I'm not buying it. Who else in the skating world but Frank would make that leap? Before he settled into coaching, he appeared in three movies as a surfboard-toting extra. Frank, who divided his time between Los Angeles and Palm Springs, was in his late seventies when we started working together, a contemporary of Kelly's who looked like he could have walked out of an Alfred Hitchcock movie and onto the ice in his fedoras.

Either way, once he mentioned the resemblance, I ran with it. Her name is Grace, after all. And what screams Old Hollywood better than a sport that in 2014 was still referring to women as "ladies," as if we all sat backstage daintily sipping tea with our pinkie fingers raised while waiting to skate?

Gracie Gold is a role that over the years I came to fully inhabit. In the same way that adults undergo an instantaneous transformation in the presence of babies—*Hello! This is my voice on helium, this is my face as Silly Putty*—I change as soon as I slip on my oversized Jackie O sunglasses. My voice rises an octave or two and my speech compresses into easily digestible sound bites like "Always wear a smile because you never know who is watching."

I had no conscious intent to erase Grace Elizabeth. The Kelly comparison was a game I played that ended up playing me. I personally never saw the resemblance. I mean, Grace Kelly was *stunning*! Much later, I would stumble upon a quote of hers that made me think we might have had more in common than I could have ever realized: "My life as a fairy tale is itself a fairy tale."

Even before I entered Frank's orbit, my transformation from spitfire to ice princess was well under way. I'd abandoned my mom's handmade outfits for the more conventional dresses that the judges and other skating officials rewarded. I'd started waxing my eyebrows regularly to give me a more polished, grown-up look. I'd begun dieting because as surely as the camera adds ten pounds to your frame, so, too, it seems, do triple and quadruple jumps. I'd learned to be more coded when expressing myself so that words didn't travel from my brain to my lips without a filter. Over the next couple of years, the metamorphosis would become complete.

I was watching a very different kind of character on the big screen—one I found much more relatable than Grace Kelly's Lisa Carol Fremont in *Rear Window*—when Frank Carroll officially entered my life. Clary Fray, a teenage half-angel, half-human warrior, was battling demons in the Shadow World when my mom's phone vibrated. We were in a darkened theater in Detroit,

Michigan, in the middle of the fantasy film *The Mortal Instruments: City of Bones,* when we were summoned to our own alternate universe.

Detroit was my way station, with Marina Zoueva and Oleg Epstein fostering me until I found permanent home ice. I spent roughly a month there, long enough to impress Marina with my work ethic. She'd never had a skater, before or since, she told me, plead for more practice ice time at a competition, like I did when she accompanied me to the U.S. International Figure Skating Classic in Salt Lake City (where I finished second). If I'm honest, all those extra sessions were my coping mechanism. They helped me tamp down my anxiety and gave me a much-needed sense of grounding when so much was up in the air.

We were less than four months out from the U.S. Championships when Scott Brown, who had choreographed some of my programs when I worked with Alex, texted Mom with the news that Frank had agreed to work with me on a trial basis. I was grateful for Scott's intervention. I assumed he was acting out of a simple desire to see me succeed. But then, given how Scott's profile soared once he started appearing with me and Frank in the kiss-and-cry area in his capacity as Frank's assistant, I'd find myself wondering if perhaps his motives had been a little more self-serving. Becoming the Grace Kelly of skating left me with a lot of jesters angling to be part of my royal court.

I'll say this for Scott. He had his work cut out for him selling me to Frank, whose initial impulse was to take a hard pass. He had heard that I was high maintenance, which surprised me, to be honest. I knew that my shouting matches with Alex could be loud, but I had no idea my voice carried all the way to Los Angeles. It speaks to the culture of skating that I was cast as the problem while the behavior of the adult, Alex, seemed to go largely unremarked upon.

Like other aspiring stars, I arrived in Los Angeles intent on reinventing myself. I was determined to mold myself into somebody more like Carly: composed, compliant, uncomplaining. If Grace Elizabeth wasn't Frank's cup of tea, what the hell, I'd become Grace Kelly. Frank had coached my idol, Michelle Kwan, and 2010 Olympic gold medalist Evan Lysacek, among others. His coaching pedigree was strong, his legacy secure. The last thing he needed or wanted was a firecracker of a kid who might explode in his hands.

I landed in Los Angeles from Salt Lake City for a two-week feeling-out period. I'd describe Frank's coaching style as detached. He revealed so little, I couldn't push any of his buttons because I didn't know what they were. It was nice for a change not to be a teenage caretaker of an adult's emotions. If I screwed up or acted out, Frank's day wasn't going to be ruined. Adjusting to Frank's coaching was like adapting to the climate of Los Angeles after living in Chicagoland. The emotional weather systems of Frank and Alex were complete opposites. I no longer had to contend with Alex's four-seasons-in-one-day volatility. In its place was Frank's pleasant, if somewhat remote, predictability.

Frank was my Professor Higgins, and I was his Eliza Doolittle. He pegged me as a skater who was technically sound but emotionally fragile. I had the skills. His job, as he saw it, was to package me in the most flattering light. To that end, he overhauled my programs, which few people would have advised with the Olympics on the horizon. My short skate to Gershwin's "Three Preludes" (or as Frank sarcastically called it, "Three Felines Fighting"): gone. He enlisted Lori Nichol, the Martha Graham of skating, to tailor a more sophisticated program that was set to a piano concerto. I kept my long program, set to Tchaikovsky's *The Sleeping Beauty,* but Frank reshaped some of it and repackaged me by insisting on new dresses and a new hairdo.

Along with revamping my looks, Frank also set about reprogramming my mind. He drummed into me that I didn't have to be perfect to win. All I had to do was be the best skater on the ice that day. I thought my head would explode. What. A. Revelation. I had always assumed that everything had to be just right when I launched myself into the air or the jump was going to be a hot mess. Frank reminded me that nine times out of ten, something's going to be a little off. The great skaters trust their internal gyroscope to make the teeny-tiny adjustments that spell the difference between salvaging a jump and screwing it up.

And if I made a mistake, so what? Frank drove home the point that no error was the end of the world. If I missed a jump, move on. Look ahead to the triple Lutz instead of dwelling on the flubbed combination. I tended to let one mistake turn into three or four. Or, worse, I'd give up, like a student who throws the test away and takes an F after she could not answer one of the first questions. If I couldn't be perfect, why bother?

Frank insisted on run-throughs at every practice, but he didn't assume I was lazy or spoiled if I started bailing on my jumps. Instead he would troubleshoot. "What are we doing, dear?" he'd say. "Are we afraid of falling? Is it something else?" Instead of kicking me off the ice after three popped jumps like Alex did, Frank would calmly tell me to recenter and carry on. I felt comfortable conveying to him that if any part of the jump didn't feel right, I didn't have the confidence to absolutely know that I could still land it cleanly. With Frank's help, I was able to let go of that thinking by reframing my perspective. Strive for land-like-a-cat consistency, jumps that were *good enough*, he said, and then let the scores fall where they may.

Muscle memory, baby. Turn off the brain and let the body take over. Frank would also insist that we do our full run-through at our first practice upon arriving at a competition venue. After we finished, he'd say, "Now you can dispel any doubts that you will fail because you just did it."

For Frank, the free skate was like a monologue. You memorize all the words until you can deliver it in your sleep. That way, when the time comes to deliver it, you can embody it—not just regurgitate it. You perform a four-minute program over and over and over in practice so that in a competition your focus isn't on each element. It's on your overall artistry.

Simple, right? Practice makes perfect. Perform your programs every day and the competitions will be a breeze. Yeah, no. The free skate really, really hurts. The lungs burn, the legs grow leaden, the arms tingle. And if you fall, pain radiates from the area that made contact with the ice. It hurts to get up. It hurts to go on. Unless you embrace the pain, which very few people can do, the physical discomfort takes a psychic toll after a while. The way I pushed through the pain was by compartmentalizing it. My mind would detach from my body, an act of dissociation that is not unlike driving on autopilot in heavy traffic and arriving at your destination without a clue that you ran three red lights to get there.

That works in practice, but in a competition, you want to be fully present. You want to feel your music, feed off the crowd. You want to be skating to your music, not through it. It's the opposite of autopilot. It's the equivalent of noting during your morning commute the sun illuminating the rolling hills and the cacophony of the schoolchildren on the playground and the smell of fresh bread drifting from the corner bakery. At competitions, I often struggled to connect emotionally to my music, or to the crowd, because I automatically went to that place of protecting myself from the pain. To that fugue state.

To keep me grounded, Frank took this tack: Imagine the worst-case scenario, he said. What if I failed to qualify for the Sochi Olympics? So what?

As Frank reminded me, he hadn't come close to making the U.S. Olympic team in his skating career and his life had turned out pretty well. I understood what he was saying, but it did nothing to stem my anxiety as the 2014 nationals drew nearer. I mean, seriously, the saying is carpe diem. When was the last time you heard someone exclaim, "Seize the long view"?

I held it together during my practice sessions but then I'd go home and lose it over my 350-calorie meal of sushi or salad. Wanna know what I called a plain bagel with three ounces of cream cheese? At 500 calories, it was a sinful splurge.

What if I let everybody down? I'd wail to my mom, who did her best to calm me. The closest I came to revealing my true feelings to Frank was when I'd say that someone's social media post really hurt my feelings. "Dear, don't read it," he'd reply. Then he'd tell me the story of how when he received hate mail, he'd stop reading as soon as he got to the nasty part, shred the letter, and throw it away. I hear you, Frank. But imagine everyone reading the hate mail at the same time that you are. That's Twitter.

To my everlasting relief, I did end up seizing the moment. I nailed my short program at the 2014 nationals to vault into first place. My 72.12 was the highest score earned by a woman at a U.S. championship under the International Skating Union's (ISU's) International Judging System (IJS). Four minutes of clean skating was all that stood between me and an Olympic berth. Before I took the ice for my long program, I stood along the sideboards in TD Garden and stared into Frank's eyes as he delivered my final instructions.

"Do your job," he said.

Right. It's worth noting what he didn't say: *Do your best. Remember to breathe. Have fun.* The time for such pleasantries had long passed. The stakes were enormous. One bobble and my dream could be deferred for another four years. Michelle Kwan's longevity made her a unicorn. Women in skating are generally like child stars in Hollywood—not exactly known for their staying power.

People assume that the Olympics are the most nerve-racking competition because the world is watching. Not if you're not there, which is why the qualifying process is so stressful. As I stood at the center of the ice waiting for the first strains of *The Sleeping Beauty,* my mind was remarkably placid. Once I reach a high level of stress, I become more calm, more unemotional, like an emergency room nurse on a particularly challenging shift. The next four minutes would determine whether I'd be known for the rest of my life as an Olympian or as just another good skater. The stakes were huge, but in that moment, the only thing I remember thinking is that I was hungry.

Hungry literally, but also metaphorically. Outside of the Olympics, there aren't a lot of other carrots to chase in skating. Contrary to what is generally believed, the top figure skaters, at least in the United States, do not as a rule become set for life financially. At events outside the Olympics, it actually costs us to represent the United States. That cap we doff during the playing of the national anthem? We have to pay for it. (The only swag we can reliably count on is the Team USA jacket.) Rare is the self-made skating millionaire. In lieu of a fortune, the Olympics are the jackpot. Qualify—or, better yet, medal—and your legacy is secure. If I faltered in the free skate, it would be devastating. Especially since the non-skating public assumed I had already secured my spot.

The selection process can be confusing because it varies from sport to sport and from country to country. In the months leading to the end of qualifying, friends and neighbors asked when I was leaving for Russia, and I was routinely introduced as an Olympian during sponsor appearances and at many public events. I appreciated everybody's support, but it was unnerving. It was even more awkward to offer up a correction, so I'd invariably smile and let the faux pas pass and pray that all the "Good luck in Sochi" greetings became a self-fulfilling prophecy. The pressure became distracting.

Fun fact: Olympic commercials are signed, sealed, and shot before many sports have chosen their Olympic teams. Which is how I wound up in a hangar-like warehouse in Los Angeles, a non-Olympian taking part in a commercial expressly tied to the upcoming Olympics. There I was applying makeup for a Visa ad as I said, "I may not look very tough, but I can accelerate faster than the guys on the racetrack, take harder impacts than a rider being thrown from a bull, and handle more g-force than a fighter pilot. But why just be extreme when you can be extremely graceful?" There I was "boarding" a Boeing 777 in my skating costume for a United Airlines commercial, twirling in the aisle and storing a piece of luggage in the overhead compartment—you know, as you do—while saying a silent prayer that I didn't become the only athlete in the shoot to be left home.

Outwardly, I appeared to be having the time of my life. I embraced the attention. I approached my interactions with the media as if I was auditioning for my own reality show. I lost count of the times I was asked how I was dealing with the pressure. Did none of the interviewers recognize that the question *was* the stressor? After the first dozen times I was asked some version of it, I decided to have fun with it. To amuse myself, I gave wildly outside-the-box answers. One that I remember was invoking one of my childhood heroines, Helen Keller. I noted that she faced a lot more adversity than I ever would. "She was able to take what she was given and make a beautiful life," I said. I added, "It just gives me chills thinking about it."

This game became another effective coping mechanism. The

more you ramble, the less you have to sit with your nerves. This Olympic season was when I added a new step to my pre-competition routine: crying jags. It was normal for me to throw up before performances (I carried breath mints in my bag for that reason). But the tears were next-level nerves. I'm talking Nicholas Sparks's *The Notebook* tears. Before my programs, I'd call Mom or Carly. Gasping for breath between sobs, I'd say, "I can't do this." They would tell me that they loved me and all that mattered was that I did my best, whatever that looked like. Just hearing their voices had a calming effect on me.

In the free skate at nationals, I was the last skater to perform, which is stressful no matter what. You have way too much time to think, and it's hard to shut out the crowd's reaction to the performances of the other skaters. When your competitors are killing it, you know. Conversely, when I glanced at the monitor and happened to see Ashley Wagner fall twice in her program, I could sense the air currents in the arena shifting to give me momentum.

I'd otherwise done my best to ignore the multiple monitors backstage as I awaited my turn. I'd eaten a bowl of regular M&M's that had been left in the designated dressing room of Scott Hamilton, who was out in the arena providing color commentary for NBC. Frank and I sat in the room for forty minutes. We passed the time talking about anything but skating. At one point Whoopi Goldberg's name came up—I wish I could remember the context—and Frank spoke about how abhorrent it was that she smoked the "devil's lettuce." Oh my God, he couldn't just say "marijuana" or "weed" like a regular person? I nearly coughed up the M&M's.

And now here I was, about to take the ice to "do my job."

I had trained hard, and well, for this moment, I told myself. As

I skated toward center ice, I said to myself, *You got this, Gracie Warrior Princess.* That was the nickname that Frank had given me. In Frank-speak, it translated to *fearless.*

Turn off the brain and allow the body to take over.

And that's exactly what I did. As the first strains of *The Sleeping Beauty* filled the rink, I became the princess awakening to her prince. I opened with a triple Lutz–triple toe combination, which I landed cleanly and with room to spare.

The Lutz is the hardest jump after the Axel, but I was so well trained that I felt extra confident in mine. I brushed the ice with my hand during an awkward triple flip, but I didn't let it undo me. With Frank's voice in my head—*Move on. Do your job*—I performed my final two triples cleanly, celebrating the last one even though I had a layback spin left to do. As I arched my back and dropped my shoulders and head toward the ice, I was actually thinking, *You just qualified for the Olympics.* If you watch the replay, you'll see me reflexively pump the air with my right fist after I nailed my last jump. It had to be involuntary because I'd never done anything like that before (and haven't since). I can only assume that becoming an Olympian triggered that primal celebration.

I knew I had skated a strong program, but to win the free skate by nearly thirteen points to earn my first national title in a rout over Polina Edmunds was beyond my wildest dreams. Fourteen months after making my senior debut, I was a national champion and Olympian. My victory came on the one-hundredth anniversary of nationals. How amazing it was, to know that my name would be forever linked with all the winners that preceded me. I was part of a through line in history that started with Theresa Weld and would continue long after I was retired.

I hadn't been perfect; I had stepped out of that triple flip. But I had held my nerve. I didn't fully appreciate at the time how rare it is to have your mind, body, and music in perfect synchronicity when it matters the most. You're lucky if you have four or five of those programs in your career, and I would have three of them in about a span of a month in 2014.

I can't say that I was overjoyed to have done my job so well. Relief was my main emotion. I was happy that I hadn't let everybody down. I do remember thinking, as the applause rained down on me and I clasped my face with my hands, that whatever happened from here on out, I was Sochi-bound. Every decision I had made in service of my skating had just been legitimized. On any CV I compiled for the rest of my life, that one word, "Olympian," would fill in the conspicuous gaps in my education and make sense of my nomadic existence.

My success turned out to be a big deal. I was coming of age at a time when the United States was desperately seeking its next ladies' headliner. The last American woman to win an Olympics singles title had been Sarah Hughes in 2002. I hadn't even started skating then. It was a shocking drought when you consider that the year Carly and I were born, 1995, skating was arguably at the height of its popularity in America thanks to its top two women, Tonya Harding and Nancy Kerrigan.

Figure skating had become front-page news before the 1994 Olympic team was finalized when Kerrigan was whacked on the knee after a practice by an assailant who then fled. The resulting injury sidelined her from nationals, but she was named to the Olympic team, anyway. So was her main rival, Harding, whose ex-husband would later be implicated in the attack.

Nancy was painted as Cinderella to Tonya's ugly stepsister. The fact that both came from blue-collar backgrounds got buried in the avalanche of news clippings about the refined and regal "artist," Kerrigan, and the rough and rebellious "athlete," Harding. One was portrayed as the white swan; the other, white trash. At the Olympics in Norway, Nancy rebounded from her injuries to win the silver and Tonya finished eighth. The competition was the most-watched Winter Olympic programming of all time in the United States.

Kerrigan was part of the streak, which started with Peggy Fleming in 1968, of eleven consecutive Olympics in which the United States placed at least one woman on the singles medals podium. The run ended in 2010 when the highest U.S. finisher was Mirai Nagasu in fourth. Four years later, two 2010 medalists, Yuna Kim and Mao Asada, were back and considered the prohibitive favorites in Sochi. A fifteen-year-old Russian upstart named Yulia Lipnitskaya was also receiving loads of attention. Eight years without an American on the podium is an eternity in our short-attention-span culture, and with cool extreme sports like moguls and aerials and half-pipe snowboarding (I'm looking at you, Shaun White) being added to the Olympic program, figure skating saw its relevance—and its audience—cratering.

And then I came along, a savior in Swarovski crystals.

It didn't matter that I went into nationals ranked outside the top ten in the world. My strong jumping and Grace Kelly vibes distracted people from my relative inexperience. I was cast as our country's brightest hope in nearly a decade to end its Olympic gold medal drought. I basked in the attention without stopping to consider that America's yearning for its next skating sweetheart was informing how I was talked about, how I was packaged. My senior international resume was pretty thin. You can't hurry experience, but with plenty of exposure people can be tricked into believing that you're an old pro, which would explain my various guest appearances on shows on NBC, the U.S. Olympic broadcast rights holder. And the ads I appeared in for the United States Olympic movement's corporate sponsors.

The pressure to be worthy of all this attention became really intense, really fast. I couldn't shake the feeling that I was cutting the line. My main rival, Ashley Wagner, was four years older and a two-time national champion, yet I was the one receiving most of the attention because of my catchy name and music-box-figurine vibes. I wasn't asking for the spotlight, but to be clear, I wasn't avoiding it. Was I selfish for going with the flow instead of pushing back against the hype? I didn't have a lot of downtime to ponder such questions. I was too busy sitting for interviews and photo shoots.

I hadn't even made the Olympic team when my "It Girl" status was established. *Sports Illustrated* decided to make me one of the magazine's four Olympics preview covers. I was in impressive company. The other athletes were the skiers Mikaela Shiffrin and Bode Miller, and the snowboarders Jamie Anderson and Arielle Gold (no relation), who appeared together. I was pictured in a stag jump. How fitting. It certainly was a leap of faith to promote someone who was only in her second year of international competition.

I was unaware that I had made the cover until we arrived in Sochi and Frank was handed a copy of the magazine by someone in the U.S. delegation. He studied it, then asked me, "Was that photograph shot on the floor of a studio?" Yes, I told him. "I'm so glad you kept your guards on," he said. "Otherwise, you would have fucked up your boots." Leave it to Frank to notice the guards on my skate blades. My eyes, meantime, were drawn to the headline, which read, "Gracie Gold as Good as . . . ?"

It was hard to escape the expectations. When I pulled up photographs in Sochi, I freaked out because they were usually attached to stories with sentences like this one in *The Daily Beast*:

"She's the adorably blond, red lipstick–wearing teen who may be America's best chance at ending a drought in ladies figure skating." Or this one in *Slate,* which described me as looking "like a blonder Disney princess whose name sounds like destiny." Or the Bleacher Report story that carried this headline: "Gracie Gold Will Thrive on Pressure to Win Gold in Sochi."

Whoa. Had none of these people heard of Yuna Kim? Mao Asada? Yulia Lipnitskaya? A day after my win at nationals, my name was the seventh-most-searched term in the United States, according to Google Trends. Having the marketing muscle of IMG no doubt helped push me into the public eye. I get it. But all the puns fit to print had something to do with it, too.

All that glitters is Gracie Gold. America's golden girl. Good as gold. Leading the gold rush. A new gold standard. Worth her weight in gold. Or my personal favorite, courtesy of the *New York Post:* "GOLD FOR IT! American Teen Poised to Resurrect U.S. Women's Skating."

I remember someone tweeting out to me, "If I hear one more Gracie Gold headline, I'm going to scream." And I was like, *Me too, bud.* It was enough to make me start wishing for a new name. Stacy Silver or Bonnie Bronze, anyone?

Then again, who was I to judge the headline writers? By the time Sochi rolled around, the hype had infected me as well. The royal blue Mini Cooper that I was driving at the time had vanity plates with just one word: GOLDN.

5

FOUR IS THE LONELIEST NUMBER

The magnitude—and majesty—of the Olympic Games didn't hit me until the Opening Ceremony, when I walked into Fisht Olympic Stadium shoulder to shoulder with others in the 200-plus-member U.S. contingent during the Parade of Athletes. The jet-engine roar of the crowd knocked me back on the heels of my black leather snow boots. The shoes were comfortable but a bit heavy for the balmy, seaside temperatures. I'll say this about the U.S. team's Ralph Lauren knit patchwork cardigans with stars—we stood out in that crowd in them. The truth? They were itchier than hell. The cream-colored cotton turtleneck sweaters and white fleece athletic pants were . . . meh. Before I dressed for the ceremony, I carefully removed the tags from the turtleneck and the pants and put them in a zippered plastic bag in case I wanted to stitch them back on at some point down the road. Like if I needed to put the outfit on eBay to cover the rent in the future. For real. Mom always taught us to plan ahead and prepare for the worst.

We were the sixty-sixth of eighty-eight nations to march into the stadium. It was overwhelming how large the venue was and, once all the athletes were inside, how small the world seemed. The ceremony lasted three hours, and by the end we were all so warm that I pictured us melting into puddles, leaving behind on the stadium floor piles of our cardigans, turtlenecks, and pants.

I cut out early to rest for the team event, which made its medal debut in Sochi. I had been chosen by our officials to represent the United States in the ladies' free skate. The new discipline featured skaters in men's and ladies' singles, pairs, and ice dance.

It was a great honor, but I was conflicted. On the plus side, it presented another medal opportunity—never a bad thing. And because the team event was in the first week, it offered me what amounted to a trial run before the ladies' singles. The extra skate could be a real confidence booster, if I skated cleanly. I was putting on a happy face, but my brain obsessed over what could go wrong. So often in my career, I'd become so overwhelmed that it would feel as if my brain short-circuited. I'd be physically present but so mentally checked out that I'd just go through the motions with a frozen smile on my face.

I really wanted that not to happen in Sochi. Team USA had the opportunity to win the first gold medal ever to be officially awarded in the team event. How often do you have the chance to be the first in history to do something? But it was really weird for all of us, as athletes in an individual sport, to have to rely on our rivals to do their jobs for us to succeed. When I was training with Alex, I hated making people run laps because I popped a jump. But this was a whole other level of accountability. Now my bad day could cost people an Olympic medal.

During my warm-up, I ignored the Olympic circles that I was skating over on the ice and pretended not to see the multiple television cameras positioned around the Iceberg Skating Palace. I chose not to dwell on the fact that in a few minutes those cameras would be beaming my performance to millions, possibly billions, of people. Thank God I was oblivious that the Russian president, Vladimir Putin, was in the audience; I might have freaked out.

I went out and did my job. I skated with a lightness that belied the magnitude of the moment in perhaps my favorite skating dress of all time. Made by Brad Griffies, my go-to designer, it was different shades of blue with a high neckline. Frank had asked him to fashion something for me that evoked Old Hollywood. He didn't need to say anything more; Brad's clients included Grace Kelly's granddaughter, so . . .

I received the second-highest score among the women, for a personal best. Only the Russian wunderkind Yulia Lipnitskaya did better, leading the Russians to the gold. Team USA secured the bronze.

It was a huge relief knowing that whatever happened the rest of the Games, I was returning home with a medal. The ladies' singles competition was at the end of the Olympics, leaving us several days to kill. The U.S. entrants—me, Polina Edmunds, and Ashley Wagner—traveled to Graz, Austria, so we could train away from the distractions of the Games. It hardly felt like we were Olympians, not when dinner every night was a quesadilla from a Hooters located near the rink where we practiced. It wasn't all work and no play, though. One day we walked from our hotel to a bridge and added a padlock decorated with our names to the thousands already adorning it.

By the time we arrived back in Sochi, I was a nervous wreck, but not about my skating. I was uptight about my fitness, by which I mean my weight, by which I mean my eating. I was paranoid about gaining a few pounds dining in the athletes' village cafeteria, anchored by free McDonald's food, and becoming "too fat to fly," as Alex was fond of saying. I was stressed about my short program because it presents so little room for error. And suddenly, after my performance in the team event, it seemed as if I was expected to make the podium.

My mom was also a wreck. She was keeping a diary for *People* magazine. In one entry, she wrote: "To manage my nerves I've been reminding myself to just accept, to let the universe unfold, and that what is supposed to happen will, that things happen the way they are supposed to. Sometimes it's great, sometimes it's painful, but it's all part of sport. I repeat over and over: 'As it should be. As it should be.'"

Security is so tight at the Olympics and our movements are so closely controlled by U.S. officials, you can't do much socializing outside the Olympic bubble, which suited me just fine. It probably was a blessing that I didn't see much of my mom during the Games because her nerves would have amplified my own.

The key in the short program was for me to get off to a strong start to settle myself. My first jump was a triple Lutz, and I felt so off in the air that the thought actually occurred to me, *Is this going to be my Olympic moment, falling on my butt?* But I fought for the landing and repeated my mantra: *Trust my training. Do my job.*

Though far from flawless, I sat in fourth place, the best among the Americans. I was more than three points ahead of one of the pre-Games favorites, Lipnitskaya, but roughly six points behind the three bunched at the top: Yuna Kim of South Korea, Adelina Sotnikova of Russia, and Carolina Kostner of Italy.

Four is the loneliest number at the Olympics. You're *so* close to the podium . . . and yet so far. I had a lot of ground to make up— too much, realistically, to earn a medal. I recognized that I was not in control of my destiny. The leaders were going to have to come back to me, and I didn't see Yuna, the defending champion and leader heading into the free skate, faltering. *Perspective, Gracie, perspective.* To calm myself, I thought of how I had been watching the Olympics four years earlier and now here I was sharing the ice with some of those same skaters. I was one of them, and maybe a kid somewhere in America would get the same thrill from watching me that I had gotten from cheering on my favorites.

In the free skate, I faced the unenviable assignment of performing right after Adelina Sotnikova, who came through with an exquisite performance. I wasn't watching, but I heard she landed a flawless triple Lutz–triple toe combination and a flurry of difficult jumps in the second half. She stepped out of a jumping combination, but it didn't hurt her because a revised scoring system was in place that rewarded attempting, if not cleanly landing, challenging elements. It also encouraged skaters to backload their programs because bonus points were given for difficult elements performed in the second half, when fatigue presumably magnified the effort. Sotnikova was seventeen, with seemingly endless reserves of stamina.

I had my headphones on and was listening to Taylor Swift and Miley Cyrus to create my own bubble. But it was impossible not to be aware that Adelina had delivered an amazing program. It honestly felt like the walls of the arena were hyperventilating as the crowd's roar reverberated off them. I stepped onto the ice while everyone was waiting for Adelina's scores. After they were announced, it was so loud that I couldn't hear Frank or the start of my own music. I just remember Frank's mouth moving like a ventriloquist's dummy. I skated to my spot and did my best to guess when my music would start. I skated well, but not perfectly. So keen was my focus, I was only vaguely aware that during a footwork sequence a clasp on the back of the neck of my costume came undone. I did four jumps with the material flapping, and thankfully I avoided flashing the world. In the back half, I fell on a triple flip, which was maddening. It was also the only time the crowd clapped for me. I dropped my right arm, as Frank had explicitly reminded me *not* to do, and the next thing I knew I was skidding across the ice on my ass.

The story I had told myself all along, to alleviate some of the pressure, was that this wouldn't be my only Olympics. I'd be back and even better in 2018. This Olympics was a trial run. My time was four years from now. Sochi was all about the experience. Blah, blah, blah. Yeah, right. It's a wonder my Barbie-doll face didn't melt from the intense emotions that I was barely managing to contain. The anger and confusion began to build as I waited for my scores in the kiss-and-cry area, which was the relief-and-regret area that day. As Frank and I listened to my scores, I had the most bizarre thought: *I would have rather been fifth or eighth than fourth.* A fifth and people would have slapped me on the back and commented on how amazing I had done. An eighth would have still been considered respectable. But a fourth was *so* close to the medals podium. Instead of dwelling on my overall success, I replayed the mistakes that cost me points that maybe could have vaulted me into third and I got mad.

Seated next to me, Frank could feel my fury rising. I vaguely remember his lips moving as he escorted me backstage. "Fourth place is respectable, Gracie. Be proud of yourself." His attempts to calm me down only riled me up. I snarled something at him, I can't even remember what. But I know what I was thinking. *Can he not simply recognize and accept my disappointment? Right after the performance, I'm in no frame of mind to hear the bright side. Can he not acknowledge the cross that every perfectionist bears— you demand that you get it exactly right, and when you don't it feels like the end of the world? It's all or nothing.*

Lots of feelings were washing over me. I was overwhelmed by

relief that I hadn't totally fucked up at the Olympics. I was overwhelmed to miss a medal by one spot. I was overwhelmed by questions from reporters about how disappointed I was to finish fourth. I was overwhelmed by the contradictory nature of my emotions.

With the benefit of time, I'd recognize that Frank was right. Fourth place at the Olympics was an incredible accomplishment. Going in, I would have been thrilled with a top-six finish. But in the immediate aftermath of my long program, when the cameras were on me and I was still breathing hard from the effort—a *losing* effort—perspective eluded me. I felt like a fraud. A deflowered America's Sweetheart. The disappointment of missing the podium was raw. I hadn't had any time to process it.

I needed to find a quiet space, a bathroom stall or unoccupied car, to lock myself in and sit with my feelings for a few minutes. Maybe scream them out. But, hello. This was the Olympics. I felt literally like the eyes of the world were on me, including the unforgiving gaze of the skating media, whose members demand sickly sweet comportment and a happy, happy face no matter what has gone down on the ice. To fall short of that is to invite articles about your ingratitude and your "shocking" attitude. In their eyes we're all athletes in pretty boxes, to borrow a phrase from one of their own, Joan Ryan. As a result, most skaters are too deathly afraid to act even remotely real, so everybody ends up sounding completely unrelatable and boring. In the absence of reliable, real, or informative reporting, speculation and gossip rush in to fill the vacuum, which makes us even less inclined to reveal ourselves and serve up our vulnerabilities on a platter in the interview area known as the mixed zone.

In Sochi, everywhere I turned a camera was pointed at me. There was no time to decompress. I had media, drug testing, the gala, the Closing Ceremony. And when the Olympic flame was extinguished at Fisht Olympic Stadium, I would be America's Sweetheart no more. What would I turn into? Not a regular teenager, exactly, but after months of photo shoots and television interviews and riffs on Helen Keller, how could I not feel a little . . . adrift?

How I wish I could time-travel back to February 20, 2014, and give that overwhelmed girl sitting next to Frank a tender talking-to. *Hey, guurrll, it's okay. Give yourself a fucking break. You did great. Be proud of yourself. Everything will look better when you've gained some distance from this five-ring carnival funhouse mirror.*

I was feeling a lot of feelings, but I couldn't begin to express to Frank what was going on. I was near the locker room entrance when Yuna's scores were announced. Adelina was also in the hallway. Upon realizing that she had won, Sotnikova rushed past me to meet up with her coach. As I walked by them, they were locked in a celebratory embrace.

As soon as the door closed behind me, I bawled my eyes out. They were tears of relief and regret. Relief that my Olympics was over and regret that the triple flip, a jump I'd executed cleanly thousands of times before, had forsaken me. I was struck by this thought: *You didn't do your job, and now you'll never know if your best would have been good enough to medal.*

I was crying even before I saw this headline courtesy of the *Daily Mail* online: "Down and Out! US Figure Skaters Polina Edmunds and Gracie Gold BOTH Fall in Final Routines as Ashley Wagner Fails to Inspire."

Ashley finished seventh. Polina was ninth. Three women in the top ten isn't exactly the end of the world. The headlines merely made it seem so. A judged sport virtually guarantees that no competition is complete without a little controversy, and sure enough, in Sochi some insiders had predicted Sotnikova's victory over Kim before either performed their long programs. Adelina always seemed to receive higher scores in her homeland than anywhere else, and the nine judges included the wife of the long-time president of the Russian Skating Federation. So when Adelina stepped out of a jumping combination and still managed to beat Yuna, who skated a clean program, it was a shock but few were surprised.

The judging is always the wild card in skating, especially at international competitions that bring geopolitical alliances into play. In this case, conspiracy theories abounded. A petition calling for an independent investigation of the results gathered more than one and a half million signatures. The scoring controversy, it turned out, was a red herring, directing everyone's attention away from Russian tampering of a much more serious nature.

So much is out of a skater's control, no matter how careful their preparation, that it can drive you crazy if you let it. That goes for parents, too. Mom was a unique skating parent in many ways. She didn't hover near the boards during a practice breathing down our coach's neck. She didn't make us drink a certain Chinese herbal tea because she heard it would forestall puberty, as the father of one skater I knew was rumored to have done. She was shockingly chill at competitions. She never demanded a coaching credential, as other parents did, so she could keep an eye on us backstage. She gave me plenty of space. She would sit in the nosebleed seats of the arena, where she could be neither seen nor heard. She didn't make me walk home or give me the silent treatment if I lost (I've known athletes who have endured worse after a poor result). Several hours after my fourth-place finish in Sochi, when I finally got to see her, she was nothing but supportive.

On the other hand, she did weigh me at home, dress me down

after bad practices, and use our skating as a way of avoiding her shitty marriage. Carly and I have turned this riddle over in our minds a lot, and we can't decide: Does the sport attract people with a few loose screws? Or does it proceed to loosen them?

All I know is that after I returned from Sochi, things went downhill fast.

6

FEEDING OUR PASSIONS, STARVING OURSELVES

I enjoy watching track-and-field competitions on television, though it makes me a little jealous when I see the contorted faces of the sprinters, their expressions of pain telegraphing the effort required to run so swiftly. In skating, we aren't afforded that luxury. It sometimes strikes me as less a sport than a magic act: Come see the pretty girl in a tiny dress execute the hardest moves possible while making it look effortless.

The sport sells an image of easy athleticism and natural beauty that is very appealing—until you know how the illusion is achieved. Few people who enjoy the sport's aesthetics are eager to be drawn into a conversation about how the skaters they love to watch stay so small or what body type is best suited to execute three and a half or four revolutions in the air in under a second. These conversations aren't encouraged because the truth about how a skater becomes world-class is not pretty.

I have non-skating friends who trudge to the gym less for fitness or fun than because they love to eat (or drink). For them, exercise is part of a simple math equation. The more calories they burn lifting weights or sweating through a hot yoga class, the more they can eat (or drink) and still button their pants. They look at my schedule—five hours on the ice, two hours in the gym, ballet classes, spin classes—and they think I have it made. They assume I must be able to eat whatever I want since I am so active.

How cute of them.

I'd venture to guess that many of us who exercise the most are actively consuming fewer calories, in general, than our more sedentary peers. That's because decades of intense exercise have turned our bodies into impressive machines that burn energy with maximum efficiency. We can do more with fewer calories. But there's also an element of control in play. Many of us are actively manipulating our metabolisms. We can't help ourselves. It's almost inevitable that the obsessive behaviors that ensure our excellence spill over into our diets. We feed our passion by starving ourselves.

It is our fault—and it isn't. Athletes and parents are misled in myriad ways: by coaches, sure, but also by a culture that conveys that thin is better. Rest in peace the age of the fleshy females of the artist Rubens's paintings, whose beauty and desirability rested in all those extra pounds. In skating, as in society, you're conditioned from a young age to believe that everything good that you aspire to achieve is contingent on how small you are. It can be as innocuous as an adult telling a child who has just finished a session and is hungry, "You don't really need those M&M's, do you?" And it can be as blatant as a coach making a weight goal a prerequisite for competing. The stress of living on the edge all the time is untenable. Self-sabotage is inevitable. Eventually you reach the point where you're like, *I'm done*, and you turn in desperation to your sworn enemy, food, for comfort.

I consider myself one of the lucky ones. I enjoyed twelve or thirteen years of carefree eating before any food compulsions kicked in. I consumed more than two thousand calories some days without giving it a moment's consideration. When I won the 2012 U.S. junior ladies' singles title, when I finished second at the 2012 World Juniors, when I placed second in my U.S. senior ladies' debut in 2013, I was on what I call a vending machine diet. I consumed whatever snacks were stocked at the rink: chocolate milk, Butterfingers, M&M's, Doritos; I wasn't picky.

Meals consisted of pasta, pizza, chicken fingers, or peanut butter and Nutella sandwiches. And because I often ate for taste, I'd end up uncomfortably full. Long live those days. I can't see them ever coming around again. Such is the food maze that I've been lost in for years. A good day now is when I supplement my bottomless-cup-of-coffee diet with one well-rounded meal.

What happened? Puberty . . . and the triple Axel. They arrived in my life at roughly the same time and, working in tandem with the culture in and out of skating, turned my physical appearance into a crisis. I was applauded for juggling three lemons in front of Jay Leno on late-night television, but no one ever wants to have a conversation about what it's like to be a teenage girl juggling the realities of her maturing body and the demands of sport. Your body develops curves and your center of gravity shifts, which change how you feel as you move through space. Add to that the challenge of coming to grips with a body you neither recognize nor necessarily relish, and which attracts attention that can be uncomfortable, and you can understand the appeal of shrinking your body to pause the whole process.

Figure skating is perhaps uniquely vulnerable to disordered eating because of the subjectivity of the judging. In the absence of a clock that objectively separates the best 100-meter runner from the rest, ice skating inevitably becomes a petri dish for insecurities.

You can skate better than everyone else but lose because your lines didn't look elegant enough, which has nothing to do with the height of your jumps or the speed of your spins. That can leave you feeling frustrated and vulnerable, but since competitors are discouraged from outwardly projecting either of these feelings—lest they come across to the judges as unrefined—they are expressed indirectly, through mental health challenges or coldness toward rivals.

From watching televised sports, I've intuited that there's a gendered difference in the discussion of weight. As my body issues intensified, people talked to and about me as if my problem wasn't with eating but with willpower, as if weight is a behavioral issue rather than a possible symptom of a mental health crisis: *You're a fat cow! No one respects you! You have no discipline! You're a joke! A clown! Snap out of it!*

I considered myself out of shape, not because I had a bad diet or mental health issues or was coming off an extended vacation, but because of some personality defect. I never thought to question the narrative until I tuned in to the telecast of a preseason NBA game and the broadcasters turned their attention to a player who was clearly carrying a few extra pounds on his frame. The analyst observed that the player needed to work himself into shape. And then the conversation moved on.

My mind was blown. How radical to hear people talk about a weight issue as if it required a change in habits, not a character makeover. Criticize the extra pounds, not the person carrying them. Fat-shaming has gone out of fashion in most corners of the culture. But in figure skating it is still practiced, albeit with euphemisms like "unfit" or, my favorite, "soft," being used in place of "fat."

You're made to feel that if things aren't going well, lose a little weight and they'll get better. This is what I mean. I'd ask Alex to critique a landing and he'd say offhandedly that my big butt wasn't helping my cause. It was confusing. I hadn't even been focused on weight. I remember asking Alex, "Are you saying I'm fat?" I was a fucking teenager weighed down by adolescence and all the changes that it triggered. I had no words to describe the heaviness I was feeling. So I asked for technical advice and got body dysmorphia because Alex didn't have the first clue what it was like to be a girl going through puberty in the spotlight. I'm well past puberty and I can't look at my ass objectively. I have to ask my boyfriend to give me his honest assessment of how I look, to tether me back to reality, because my grip on the truth is shaky when it comes to my physical appearance.

All the literature on trauma makes clear that when faced with shame, the brain reacts the same as if confronting a physical danger. In my mind, the discomfort of withholding food from my body was less scary than the hurt of being rejected, as I saw it, by a man I loved like a father. If Alex said I needed to lose five pounds, I was determined to lose ten, so he'd be doubly pleased and impressed.

I started to keep track of calories the way others monitor their steps, with an app. By no means am I promoting this—in fact, my hope is that people will do as I say and not as I did and avoid this app, MyFitnessPal, which for me and many other women I know served as the gateway to disordered eating. I set a ceiling of one thousand calories and whittled my intake from there until I was subsisting on less than five hundred calories a day. Looking back, I can see that my behavior was yet another coping strategy. The time I spent obsessing over how many calories I consumed was time not spent obsessing over the Olympics.

I developed a few weight-loss hacks involving food substitutions. I'd take a favorite dish—lasagna, for example—and I would research the lowest-calorie version of it: spaghetti squash pasta (31 calories versus 131 for regular pasta), tofu instead of ricotta cheese (78–88 calories versus 174), dairy-free cheese substitute (plant-based mozzarella is 80 calories for one-quarter cup versus 90 calories for regular mozzarella), and sugar-free marinara sauce (70 calories per serving versus 80). The sauce trade-off may sound like small tomatoes, if you will, but it's actually torture for me because I'm so fond of regular spaghetti sauce I've been known to eat spoonfuls of it straight from the jar.

Exhausting, right? Always evaluating food in terms of calories instead of taste turns eating into calculus.

I hated calculus.

I weighed myself every damn day. How I felt about myself became quantifiable. It was based on the number I saw on the scale. Whereas before I had judged my worth on the flawlessness of my programs, I now began to value myself based on the severity of my caloric restriction. My mantra became, *If I don't eat today, everything will be great. If I'm thin enough, my problems will disappear.* An eating disorder is a perfect disease for a control freak. It affords you the illusion that you alone hold the reins to your life. You can manage it through the number of calories you consume.

The issue was that my body craved fuel because of the energy I was expending in training. If I didn't eat, I was physically weak. If I gave in to my body's demands and supplied the nutrition it needed, I considered myself morally weak; I had lacked the strength of character necessary to push through my hunger.

When I finished second at my first senior nationals, I was a super-lean but not malnourished size four, with a tiny upper body and chest and muscular thighs. When I looked around, I noticed for the first time that I was surrounded by girls in size two or zero costumes. Once opened, my eyes could not unsee all the rail-thin figures in my midst.

My obsession with thinness led me down some scary rabbit

holes online. Early on, I searched "How to be anorexic" and stumbled upon forums that contained helpful suggestions on how to start, and sustain, starvation. I'd allow myself one cheat day on the weekends, usually Saturday, to make my days of deprivation more doable and also to deflect attention from my lack of eating the rest of the week. I'd dine out with friends or family and/or bake and not keep track of calories, which gave me the outward appearance of normalcy. Other than that, I was super-disciplined. There were days in the months leading up to the 2014 U.S. Championships when I allowed myself one apple or a single tomato per meal.

I used to skip meals regularly and on those rare occasions when somebody noticed and called me out on it, I'd say that I had been so busy I forgot to eat. Yeah, no. I wasn't restricting my caloric intake to "meals" that consisted of a 60-calorie skinny vanilla latte or a 57-calorie apple or a 33-calorie tomato or a 281-calorie cup of Greek yogurt because I had lost my appetite or didn't have time to eat a proper meal. I was hungry most of the time.

It's exhausting to live every day when you have a complicated relationship with something that you need to survive. Unless you've been there and done that, it's hard to make sense of it. So many people would say to me, "What do you mean you can't eat? Look at all this food." It was like saying to an asthmatic, "What do you mean you can't breathe? Look at all this air."

In the six months before my Olympic debut, I shed nearly ten pounds and lost some height and power on my jumps but gained quickness and consistency, which were really beneficial. As an added bonus, I was showered with compliments on my appearance. I was starving myself and people fell over themselves praising me: "You look fantastic! You look so fit! You could be a model!"

That's the tricky part about eating disorders in skating. As you advance deeper into your teens, to continue to progress it's almost essential to have one. Thinner people have longer lines. The challenge is to walk the tightrope line between being strong enough to perform the toughest elements but also light enough for the toughest elements to be easy to perform. Get too strong and your musculature will slow you down and hamper your flexibility. Grow too lean and your body won't have the strength or energy required to train—or, ultimately, if you take it too far, to exist. And if your growing bones and tendons snap under the stress because you're denying yourself the proper nutrients, that's what painkillers and smelling salts are for.

The Russians aren't dominating women's skating because they're taking diet pills. But after losing to Sotnikova in Sochi, I was no longer controlling my eating. My eating was controlling me. I resisted having dinner with coaches or other skaters. I didn't want them to catch on to my disordered eating. It was obviously harder to dodge Mom and Carly since we were together all the time. I'd get around it as best I could. I'd say I had eaten earlier, or I hid food in napkins in my pockets to discard later. What I didn't understand at the time was that in shying away from others at mealtimes, I was showing my hand. The avoidance of social eating was a red flag.

Or it ought to have been.

I remember confiding in a few people about my unhealthy fixation on food only to hear, "You look good." Or "You don't look sick." Their responses confirmed what I already had internalized: You're not too skinny until you almost disappear. A skater I trained with endured a lengthy hospital stay to treat her eating disorder and has to wear a heart monitor every time she works out or skates to guard against her weakened heart giving out on her. She had to nearly die before anybody realized that she was dieting herself to death. It's as if the sport has conditioned us to normalize our disordered eating.

The pressure to be lean has only increased since I burst onto the world stage, as athleticism has been prioritized more and more over artistry. Scoring changes now reward the big jumps that are best executed by the smallest people. Why is no one confronting a sport that outwardly rewards a body type that's more heroin chic than healthy?

We're allowed—and in many cases, encouraged—to have a dysfunctional relationship with food for the duration of our elite careers with the tacit approval of our coaches. And if our dysfunctional relationship with food—let's call it what it is, an act of self-harm—ends up shortening our elite careers, oh, well. There are plenty of other prospects in the pipeline. *Next!*

Does that not strike anybody else as insane? If you're painfully thin but you're skating well, it's not a problem. But what if you were abusing meth or prescription pills instead of food but somehow skating well? Would the calculation be the same?

I caution against considering that question too long. It might force you to change forever how you look at the sport.

7

LOOKING DOWN ON MYSELF

The Winter Olympics take place every four years. Olympic athletes might fall off the public radar in between, but our responsibilities don't vanish with the spotlight. We still have rent and utilities to pay. Food and gas to buy. Fees for coaching, ice time, travel, skates, costumes, choreography. After Sochi, it's not like I could take my bronze medal and chop it into pieces to pay my bills.

In the weeks immediately after I returned from Russia, I was able to trade on my Olympic accomplishment to enjoy some surreal experiences. I established a casual friendship with Taylor Swift, whose songs were part of my favorite playlist at the time. She happened to see the telecast of my skate in the team event and afterward she tweeted, "Just googling when I can watch @GraceEGold skate in the Olympics next . . . How adorable and lovely is she?!" I was so excited. Then, a couple of days later, she followed me on Twitter (I had been following her for a while). I sent her a direct message thanking her for the tweet and for following me. I told her she was my hero and music idol. Taylor replied and we began a correspondence. Then Taylor sent me her cellphone number and we switched to texting.

Several weeks after I returned from Sochi, I was in New York for an ice show. Taylor was in New York, too, and she invited me to her Tribeca loft to make chocolate chip cookies from scratch. I wrapped up those fabulous cookies and brought them with me to an ice show on Long Island that I was appearing in the next night. I left them on the snacks table for the skaters. I explained that I had made them with "a friend." Taylor came to the show. I was so delighted. She joined us backstage afterward, and when she spied the crumbs that remained from the batch of cookies, she cooed, "Oh, did you guys like the cookies that Gracie and I made?" Everybody snapped their heads to look at me. Their facial expressions were priceless.

We stayed in touch, and the following December, she texted me out of the blue and asked if I was in Los Angeles. I said I was because I was preparing for the 2015 nationals. "What are you doing tomorrow?" she asked. I told her I was skating in the morning but had the rest of the day free. She explained that she was organizing a day trip to Catalina Island with a few friends. She asked if I wanted to come. "Um, YES!" I said. After skating, I drove to the coast, met her friends, which included the singer Lorde, and we made a boat crossing to Catalina, had lunch and ice cream cones for dessert, then sailed back to the mainland.

I'd never confuse Catalina for Sochi (except for the weather, which wasn't all that different in December). And yet when I think of special memories from the Olympics, it's not any interactions at the athletes' village that stand out or even the competition itself. It's wonderful, whimsical days like my boat trip with Taylor and her gal squad, made possible only because she saw me on TV skating on our sport's biggest stage.

That was a great day, but the months after the Olympics were filled with many more terrible, horrible, no-good, very bad days. A post-Olympics debt comes due that nobody really talked about in 2014. It was so common, it had a name: the post-Olympic blues. From the time I finished second at the 2013 nationals to insinuate myself into the Sochi conversation, I had channeled all my energies into making that U.S. team. It was on my mind every single minute of my every waking hour. I returned from Russia and it was like . . . *now what?*

I experienced a huge letdown. I wondered how and where I was going to find the desire to keep going. I was eighteen years old and when I wasn't baking cookies or sailing with Taylor or appearing on the red carpet at big events, I was entertaining some profoundly disturbing thoughts: *What happens next? What will the rest of my life look like? Was Sochi as good as it'll get? Who will I be if I'm not a competitive skater?*

I was hurtling toward a quarter-life crisis. Too young to legally drink to my success. Too old to blindly believe that my best skating days were ahead of me. I had a number of endorsement contracts, including with CoverGirl, Nike, Red Bull, and Smucker's. I was near my peak earning power, I was miserable, and few people were sympathetic. I heard a lot of some variation of *"What do you mean, you're confused/depressed/sad? I just watched you in the Olympics!"*

I was in a weird space. It seemed as if the world knew me, but nobody really saw me. I was the Olympic skater in everybody's eyes. Grace Elizabeth, inasmuch as she still existed, was invisible. Gracie Gold was an object of desire, envy, adoration, while Grace Elizabeth slowly slipped into nothingness.

My dilemma was this: How could I fix a malaise that nobody else saw? Increasingly, taking a shower became a monumental task, not because I didn't care about my hygiene but because I did not care about existing. I thought making the Olympics would solve all my problems. But I came back from Sochi with the same body dysmorphia, the same self-hatred, the same tangled family dynamics, all of which were exacerbated by my higher public profile. A chasm opened between how I looked at myself and how others saw me. A great example was the Malibu High student who invited me to his senior prom in a video that went viral on social media. "Watching you skate has made me realize how perfect we are for each other. . . . You're gorgeous. My mom thinks I'm pretty." He laid it on thick. "The Olympic judges got it wrong. You're the only gold I see."

It was a sweet gesture, but I couldn't go because I had a post-Olympic skating tour scheduling conflict. But then the producers of a cable television entertainment show arranged a surprise (for me, anyway) meet-cute moment with my would-be prom date during an already-scheduled interview. As I acquired a few stalkers, including one who hacked my personal email, I would come to question the propriety of so many boundary-crossing experiences that were all in a day's work for me around this time, starting with, but not limited to, an adult television producer acting as a matchmaker for a teenager for the sake of ratings. I wondered why I was expected not only to allow myself to be exploited in this way but also to be *grateful,* because figure skating can't buy that kind of publicity. *You want to set me up with a perfect stranger who for all anybody knows could be unhinged? Why, yes, please! And thank you!*

And of course, there was the faceless critic lurking in the recesses of my mind, reminding me that the Malibu student was infatuated with Gracie Gold. Grace Elizabeth no doubt would have been a massive disappointment to him. I was trained to sell a performance on the ice, and after the Olympics that behavior bled into my life. I became super-invested in everybody believing that I was a sound-bite-delivering doll living her best life because I didn't want to disappoint people. I was convinced that people would not find the real me likable.

In the fall of 2014, I injured my left foot in practice the week before the NHK Trophy in Japan. I was still able to skate, though it hurt like hell. I had the foot X-rayed at an urgent care center and, thankfully, there was no visible fracture. I was told I probably had tendinitis, and tendinitis is the common cold of sports, so off to Japan I went.

Somehow, I still managed to win both the short program and free skate. I became the first American woman to claim that title. It turned out that I competed with a stress fracture that didn't show up on the X-ray. Looking back, I'm not surprised that I had no clue of the extent of the injury until I had a CT scan and MRI after the competition. My powers of dissociation were so well practiced by then, it felt like much of the time I was outside my body looking down on myself.

Injuries are bound to happen when you're balancing on ice. But my eating habits heightened my vulnerability. When I think back to the months after the Sochi Olympics, what I remember is how hectic my days were and how haphazard my diet became. I was essentially doing just enough training to get by in between traveling for public appearances on behalf of my sponsors and for U.S. Figure Skating and the United States Olympic and Paralympic Committee (USOPC). Because I wasn't back in hardcore training and I was eating on the run, I put on fifteen pounds (call it the banquet-circuit fifteen). I'm sure the combination of restricting my diet for a year, followed by eating all the delicious pastries and snacks in television green rooms and on sponsors' catering tables, followed by frantically restricting my eating again, contributed to the fracture. It was, in some manner, a self-inflicted injury.

With my national title defense less than two months away, officials from U.S. Figure Skating and the USOPC recognized that I was in a full-blown physical crisis and sought to help me. I was steered to a top-notch orthopedist who supervised my rehabilitation, and a bone stimulator device was sent to my home to accelerate my healing.

By the time my left foot was healed, I had roughly two weeks to prepare for nationals. Given how little ice time I had logged, I was satisfied with my second-place finish behind Ashley Wagner in Greensboro, North Carolina. She and I were in the midst of a five-year stretch in which we took turns winning the ladies' title. The media made us out to be rivals along the lines of Tonya and Nancy, but it was a forced narrative that reporters ran with for page clicks and content. The only thing that was said about us that was truthful was that we didn't much care for each other. We were different people with different temperaments vying for the same crowns. That's it. End of story.

Ashley said I pushed her to get better, and I'd agreed that she did the same for me. She was a tough competitor. I hated when she won, but there was no shame in losing to her.

From the outside, though, my result was seen differently—not as a small measure of success but as a failure to defend my title. I let others, no matter how uninformed, trigger my self-loathing. An acceptable result, when seen through these outsiders' eyes, became unsatisfactory. It breathed into being the version of myself that I now call "Outofshapeworthlessloser," a faceless bogeyman who made herself at home in my head. It was a pathology of my personality that lay dormant for many years before entering a period of rapid growth in the years after my Olympic debut.

Outofshapeworthlessloser would lead me down some desolate dead ends in search of fixes for the "flaws" in my physical appearance. Nobody around me seemed to seriously question why I was invested in being a world-class athlete yet wouldn't fuel my body.

Not only did I deny myself basic nutrition, but I also took other extreme measures that could have inflicted permanent damage. For example, laxatives became part of my weight management around this time. When I couldn't deprive my body another day, I'd go to the opposite extreme and consume a huge meal only to have my stomach puff out like yeast dough. Because of my erratic eating habits, my gut health was horrid. I hated feeling bloated, so one day in desperation I got in my car and steered it to the nearest drugstore in search of relief. I poked around the aisles for an over-the-counter stool softener. That's the shorthand version of how I became hooked on laxatives. When I arrived in Shanghai for the 2015 World Championships, my pursuit of a medal took a temporary backseat to my pursuit of laxatives.

I was consuming eight to ten pills a day by the time I arrived in China. That became a problem when I realized I had left home without enough of a supply to get me through the trip. I freaked out. If the stakes hadn't been so high, it could have been the setup for a bad joke: *A figure skater walks into a Shanghai pharmacy, shitting herself because she can't find laxatives . . .*

China is notorious for counterfeit drugs and weak regulations. You can't be sure of the accuracy of the listed ingredients, which is why I couldn't take a chance. No way was I going to risk failing a drug test for some unknown banned substance that I hadn't meant to ingest. I was too embarrassed to ask a team doctor for laxatives. My mother had accompanied me on the trip and she was accustomed to running errands for me, like returning to the hotel to get something I left behind or collecting a coffee for me when I needed a midday pick-me-up. So I leaned on her to ask the doctor for the laxatives. She said they were for Carly because she didn't want to invite any scrutiny of my practices, and Carly was furious when she found out.

After replenishing my supply, I proceeded to figuratively crap all over the ice in my short program. I was in eighth place going into the free skate. I delivered the second-best long program to salvage a fourth-place finish, one spot ahead of Ashley. With overuse, the efficacy of the laxatives waned, a problem solved by turning to other drugs, including a few whose main purpose was to treat diabetes but whose side effects included weight loss.

Despite all the pills that I was consuming in place of food, my skating stayed on track. When the next season began, I finished second to the Russian Evgenia Medvedeva at Skate America in Milwaukee. The following month I competed in the Grand Prix event in France, the Trophée Éric Bompard. It was held November 13–15 in Bordeaux, a two-hour train ride from Paris. It was the rare occasion in which I nailed my short program and everybody else faltered. My lead over the Russian Yulia Lipnitskaya going into the free skate was more than seven points. The title was mine to lose. I returned to the hotel and Mom was combing out my hair as the television played in the background when, suddenly, the screen filled with scenes of chaos. That's how we learned of the coordinated attacks by terrorists across Paris. One of the targets was a soccer stadium. It was terrifying. My first thought was, *What are they going to hit next?* My nerves about the competition gave way to anxiety about our safety.

I was making the two-block walk from the rink to the arena the next day when my cellphone buzzed. It was Frank. "Hello, dear," he said. "They've canceled the rest of the event. Congratulations on your second Grand Prix title." Frank's words stopped me in my tracks. My first reaction was, *Yay, me! I won!* followed quickly by, *Oh, shit. This is terrible. I won only because more than a hundred people died and hundreds of others were injured.*

It was one of my biggest victories, but I felt sad and numb. I hadn't earned the title. It had been handed to me by default. I had done half the work for the whole enchilada.

After my strong showing in the fall, I came to the 2016 nationals ready to win. My short program was so on-brand for me—a real crime scene of a skate. Those two minutes and fifty seconds are like a true-false test where you tick off the required jumps, spins, and step sequences: Triple jump out of footwork, yes or no? Lay back spin, yes or no? I'd be figuratively holding my breath the whole time. One mistake and you were sunk. And I made multiple mistakes.

The free skate feels more like an essay exam. I had time to breathe and room enough to express the full scale of my athleticism, choreography, and musicality. So even though it was longer and harder (maybe *because* it was longer and harder), I much preferred it.

I knew I could not mess up a single element. The math did not portend a favorable outcome. I needed a score five points higher than my personal best to surpass Polina Edmunds. Skating directly before me, she had delivered an impeccable performance.

The good news was, there was no ambiguity to my situation. I knew exactly what I had to do: skate perfectly. I remember waiting for my music to start, thinking that now would be a clutch time to summon one of those magical performances where everything clicks and you feel completely in the zone.

The opening notes of my *Firebird* music started, and unbelievably, as I was picking up my right skate after flapping an arm a few seconds into my program, my foot fishtailed. It was probably imperceptible to most everybody else, this split-second lapse in concentration. Imagine a basketball player tripping on his way to the free-throw line. That's what it was like. Weirdly, that bobble snapped my mind to hyperattention.

From that point on, I skated beautifully. With each jump, my intensity level increased. I wasn't launching myself into the air so much as floating heavenward. I was leading with my chin. I know my edges were digging into the ice, but, honestly, by the end it felt as if I wasn't even touching the ground. I had never more fully inhabited the Gracie Gold persona. After I cleanly landed my final triple, a triple Salchow, my smile was incandescent. "Amazing!" Frank said as I stepped off the ice. Like a record stuck in a groove, he kept repeating himself. *Amazing! Amazing! Amazing! Amazing!*

To this day, Frank says that my skate that night was one of the greatest performances by any athlete with whom he worked.

Everything just lined up so perfectly at exactly the right time. It was the absolute best I'd ever skated, and I truly believed the best was yet to come. All I had to do was keep my eating under control and my skating would take care of itself. If I could continue starving myself, the world would be mine.

The World Championships were next. They were taking place in the United States. Not just on home soil but in my hometown, Boston. Not only where Carly and I were born but also where I won my first national title to qualify for the Olympics. The script couldn't have been written any better. The stage was beautifully set for me to become the first U.S. skater to win a World Championships singles title since Kimmie Meissner in 2006.

There was extra pressure with the event taking place in the

United States. Pressure can corrode your nerves like battery acid, but I honestly felt pretty chill. Confident, even. I told reporters at nationals that I was going to be on the medals podium at the World Championships. I didn't even bother to couch my prediction.

I was right. The World Championships would be a defining moment for me. It was the competition where Gracie Gold, as the world knew her, ceased to exist.

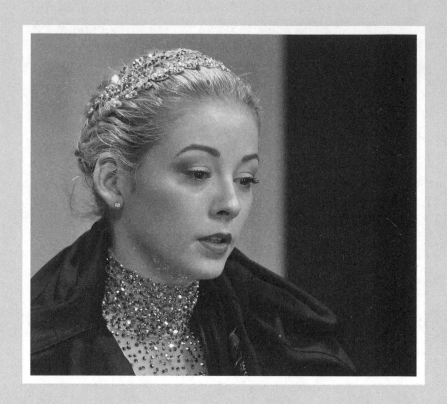

OUTOFSHAPE-
WORTHLESSLOSER

PART THREE

Sometimes good things fall apart so better things
can fall together.

—Attributed to Marilyn Monroe

8

HAUTE MESS EXPRESS

There I stood on home soil, poised to win a World Championships medal, possibly a gold. It was April 2, 2016, and I was in first place heading into my *Firebird* free skate, the same program that I had performed almost flawlessly at nationals a few weeks prior. Could I conjure another four minutes of flow and flight and pure delight? At my best, I was an addict craving that adrenaline rush. At my worst, I was a perfectly accessorized packet of anxiety in fight-or-flight mode. I never could be sure which me would show up. I felt enormous pressure to give American skating fans a gold medal moment, as Michelle Kwan had at the 2003 World Championships in Washington, D.C. The 2.45-point lead I took into the free skate was nice, but it wasn't insurmountable. The perfectionist inside me was on high alert.

In the free skate, Evgenia Medvedeva, a sixteen-year-old Russian who was making her World Championships senior debut, produced the skate of her life. She performed way better than she had in the short program in France a few months earlier, and received the highest score ever recorded in the ladies' competi-

tion, 150.10. So incredible was her skate, I would have had to record a score ten points higher than what I earned at nationals in
the long program to pass her. I didn't have to do the math in my
head to know that I had to pull out all the stops. Another Russian, Anna Pogorilaya, nailed her program just before me. I knew
even before her scores were announced, from the cheers that
rocked the arena, that the other ladies had come to play.

It was my turn to respond. To *compete*. To *attack*. Instead,
thirty-four seconds into my program, I inexplicably fell on the
second jump of my opening combination, a triple toe loop. I had
plenty of height on it and my mechanics were sound right up
until I returned to the ice on legs tighter than a botoxed face and
lost my balance. My right hand grazed the ice, and the next thing
I knew I was in the yoga crab pose. In the commentary booth,
Tara Lipinski let out an involuntary gasp. As I picked myself up,
Johnny Weir said gravely, "In a performance where Gracie needs
ten points above her personal best, starting off with a fall is not
the most encouraging way."

No shit! My mind was reeling, but my muscle memory took
over. Triple loop. Double Axel. Double Axel–triple toe–double
toe. Triple flip–double toe. A triple Lutz that I turned into a double. Triple Salchow. I reeled off the rest of my jumps like a zombie
Barbie, cleanly landing them but sealing my fate with my Lutz
mistakes. I had protected myself against failure instead of charg-
ing. Instead of seizing the moment, I had let the moment seize
me. I knew the second my music stopped that I had blown it.

All I wanted to do was rush off the ice and lock myself in the
bathroom. But of course, figure skating doesn't allow that. One
of the strangest—and, often, cruelest—customs of figure skating
is the bows you have to take after each performance. Imagine:
You've just fucked up royally. Your worst nightmare has come

to pass. But instead of disappearing behind a thunderhead of shame, you now have to stand at center ice and curtsy to the judges who are marking you down as you acknowledge them; to the crowd who has just witnessed your biggest failure in person; to the folks at home who gasped and then grabbed a handful of mixed nuts while you, after starving yourself for two years, hit the ice so hard that you'll have a bruise in the morning. There you are, mouthing the words "Thank you; thank you so much" through a stiff smile, while your dreams—like all the stuffed animals being thrown by eager ten-year-olds in the stands—crash land around you. As I skated off the ice, Journey's "Don't Stop Believin'" filled the arena. Well played, Mr. DJ. However sincere the intent, the music choice struck me as pure mockery.

Seated next to Frank in the kiss-and-cry area, I could feel disappointment radiating from his pores. I wanted to swipe that black fedora from atop his head and stomp on it. In that cramped space, we didn't make eye contact. Our bodies didn't touch. I put on a brave face, smiling vacantly, vaguely aware of Scott Brown, seated on my other side, patting me on the back consolingly, and wondering all the while if NBC really needed to be *that* up close and personal on what was shaping up as the most tragic moment of my skating life.

My technical scores were not great. My artistic marks were slightly better. I dropped to third, behind the two Russians, whom I had to awkwardly share a room backstage with while the final competitor, Ashley Wagner, skated her face-off. Afterward, a TV camera was trained on me while I waited to hear if I was going to fall off the medals podium. I kept my head down and furiously texted Carly, who was somewhere in the building. I had nothing to tell her. I was just tapping my keyboard to have something to do. Ashley's scores made it official: An American had made the podium, but it was not me in third. It was Ashley in second. The U.S. medal drought was over, but my misery was just beginning.

I smiled for the camera, my frozen grin meant to convey, *Yay, America!* I was in a daze. *If* I had skated like I did every damn day in practice, I would have won a medal. How could I have been so tight when I was so ready for that moment?

My mask never dropped. But as a media volunteer escorted me through several TV stops and a print media scrum backstage, my disappointment showed.

I stopped to talk to a Portuguese broadcaster, who asked, "In your own words, what's your feelings now?"

"I mean, I'm really sad and I'm really embarrassed, and I feel really ashamed of how I skated and how I tried to represent my country. It just is a really, really terrible moment for me and my skating. There's not much to say. Just during the course of this week, I lost a lot of shape. And I just couldn't keep up with my expectations and with the other skaters. I still have hopes for the 2018 Olympics, but we'll really have to step back and reevaluate what's realistic for my future in skating."

Clearly taken aback, the man asked, "Aren't you a bit harsh with yourself?"

"Um, I mean, if you look at the skating and the quality of the skating and the scores, I just feel it's accurate. And it's what every-body else is going to say anyway."

The media volunteer looked away. She would later say that it pained her to see me lashing myself with my words. At the next three broadcasting stops, it was more of the same.

"Obviously, I couldn't motivate myself and get going. It just shows I'm not up there with the rest of the world . . ."

"It was a very, very unfortunate and sad experience. This is probably my only shot at really being at the top in the world . . ."

"I feel sorry for Boston and the United States because I feel like I

let them down when they needed me the most. I'm sorry to every-
body that supported me that I couldn't deliver. I'm really sad and
I'm really embarrassed."

From stop to stop I went, dry-eyed and flat-voiced, an actor on
autopilot. The media volunteer grew increasingly alarmed. She'd
never heard someone talk with such self-loathing. She would
later say she wanted to shake some sense into me, get right up in
my face and say, *Don't talk that way about yourself. You're still one*
of the best in the world.

She dutifully recorded my answers at each stop on a digital
recorder. She was responsible for transcribing my interviews to
distribute to the media. But her protective instincts kicked in.
She wasn't a trained journalist and didn't pretend to be. She suspected that what she was doing was not exactly aboveboard, but
she left out the worst of my comments. She didn't want my words
to become catnip for insensitive reporters.

So shook was the media volunteer, she said, she tracked down
my agents afterward. She warned them that I was not well. Something must be terribly wrong for me to speak of myself in such
a disparaging fashion, she told them. Her message was not received as she had hoped. A few weeks later, I was back on the
road as one of the headline performers in Stars on Ice, a figure-
skating extravaganza produced by IMG, the company that represented me.

I've given a lot of thought to this period in my life, pondered
what I could have, or should have, done differently to slow my
slide. One thing that would have helped a lot is if the people
around me, starting with Frank, hadn't acted as if my career had
died out there on the TD Garden ice.

Frank would blame the drop-off in my performance from the
short to free skates on my eating habits. His consternation was
rooted in my parents regaling him with tales of our fancy Italian

dinner the night before in Boston's North End. It didn't matter that I don't recall consuming more than a few bites of my spaghetti Bolognese before pushing away my plate. On some level, I must have accepted his explanation for my failure to medal as fact, because when I hit the mixed zone where the world's print and digital reporters were gathered, I repeated over and over that I had "lost some shape." There were echoes in Frank's explanation of the days when Alex would describe me as a world-beater one day and a fat cow the next.

The truth? I didn't lose my shape. My family was what was coming apart. And I was just so fucking sad about it. It was a totally normal reaction to what was going on, but in figure skating there's no room for anything but those happy, happy faces.

I'm sorry if I had a hard time focusing on the beautiful music when I never knew from one day to the next which way the family friction would rub. I admit that Tara wasn't wrong when she called out my lack of confidence in the commentary booth. What she failed to get right was why I was a mental mess. She said: "When I was talking to Frank, he said, 'She should be a world champion.' He said, 'Day in and day out she's so consistent. Never misses. But when she goes out in a competition and lets her mind get in the way, it's maddening.'"

Frank looked at me and saw someone disproportionately blessed with beauty, talent, and a supportive family. In his eyes, I lacked nothing. From his vantage point, I seemed almost disdainful of the gifts I'd been given. He didn't grasp that my eating habits and fluctuating weight were symptoms of what was wrong, not the root causes. If he couldn't understand the source of my self-loathing, it's because he never scratched beyond the surface for answers. My life didn't strike him as difficult or complicated. He had a hard time mustering sympathy for someone who appeared to have it all, yet seemed hell-bent on sabotaging her success. His reserve created a space between us, even when we were sitting thigh to thigh. I could never bridge that space. I could never shake the feeling that he could take me or leave me. Or, worse, that he never really knew me.

It was obvious that I was fragile, but nobody drilled down very deep to understand why. It was easier to blame my eating habits or my mental fragility because those things could conceivably be fixed. They're much easier to address, at least on the surface, than a broken family, which is terribly hard to mend.

My behavior got blamed, not my environment, because when behavior is the problem, it offers the promise that we're all just a few self-help steps from a world and a life free of pain, criticism, and failure. Instead of asking questions, people gave me a wide berth, which left me feeling incredibly alone, a castaway on the Island of Misfit Skaters. People say that the World Championships in Boston crushed me. That I never recovered from that fourth-place finish. Yeah, no. The competition itself wasn't what sent me rolling downhill like a snowball, picking up speed and size as I almost fell off the face of the earth. The real trauma was what happened next. How people responded to that fourth-place finish was the problem. In my time of need, I struggled to find emotional support.

So many people were invested in my success: my family, Frank, U.S. Figure Skating, everybody I left behind in Springfield, Missouri, and Illinois, my tens of thousands of social media fans—which meant that my failure wasn't just my disappointment. It was theirs, too. I had let everyone down and no one knew what to say to comfort me. They felt sorrow, or pity, but since those aren't emotions that are suitable to express in skating, they said nothing. Or they offered pithy words of comfort.

The day after the free skate, I talked with U.S. Figure Skating's senior director of high performance, Mitch Moyer. We met at his insistence. He said he was genuinely concerned after my devastating free skate. He told me he cared about me as a person. I'm sure he meant well, but the conversation rang hollow. I had never been able to relate to the older, mostly white gentlemen overseeing our sport. They were like distant uncles, or worse, stand-ins for my dad—awkward to talk to, impossible to confide in. They didn't seem to understand that trust is not automatic; it isn't conferred with a fancy title. It's earned over time, through dozens of small interactions that indicate a genuine concern and caring. I liken it to the work acquaintance who reaches out after a tragedy and says, "I'm here for you." That's sweet, but if our relationship is superficial, I'm not going to want to bare my soul to you.

In that moment I didn't want to be rescued. I wanted to be heard. Supported. Accepted for the disappointed state that I was in rather than told to accentuate the positives. I could have attempted to articulate this to Mitch, but it felt like too much work. Also, it was one of those situations made for this maxim: "If I have to explain this to you, you're never going to get it." How could I begin to make him understand that I was physically present on the ice during the free skate but mentally out of it, my brain so awash in stress that I was out there just trying to survive?

And so I resorted to sarcasm instead. It's always been a very handy device to save me from having to confront my real feelings. I told Mitch, "This conversation is why American women are not consistently on the podium, why the Russians are consistently beating us. They would have thrown me to the curb after that free skate last night."

I wasn't wrong. I must give the Russians grudging respect for one thing: They don't pretend their athletes are anything but cogs in a machine. They may be brutally obvious about it, but at least everyone is clear what the priorities are: medals over the health and well-being of their athletes. U.S. Figure Skating officials wanted us to believe that we're one big caring family when their actions with me over the years suggested the relationship was much more transactional. I make them look good, they'll make me look good.

It pains me to consider the dozens of athletes in the pipeline behind those of us grabbing the headlines whose lives also totally revolve around skating, who have left their families to train and are receiving scant compensation and even less attention from this supposedly caring and nurturing organization. The Roy children in the HBO Max series *Succession* had nothing on the dysfunctional family that was U.S. Figure Skating during this time. I stumbled upon a proverb during one of my rabbit-hole internet sessions that knocked me back in my chair: "The trees fooled themselves into believing the axe was their friend because its handle was made of wood." In the U.S. Figure Skating scenario, the athletes are the trees, and they believe the organization is their friend because it's filled with ex-skaters, coaches, and judges.

The point I was too overwhelmed to artfully make to Mitch was this: If you're not going to make the investment over time to get to know us as people, we might as well be cogs in your high-performance machine. You can't act like we're family if there's no bonding. They couldn't genuinely care about me because they didn't genuinely know me.

In the days and weeks after the competition, a suffocating blanket of resignation settled over me. Maybe I was being paranoid, but I couldn't shake the feeling that I had failed in the clutch, creating a permanent stain on my record. I was never what you'd call a consistent performer, but I could always be counted on to pull through, in the long program especially, when it really, really mattered. The higher the pressure, the more likely I was to crush it. Until that point, I saw myself—and I believe others did as well—as the Comeback Kid. To not pull through when it counted was crushing to me. If I wasn't the Comeback Kid, who was I? Another pretty face with talent? The pretty face was given to me in the birth roulette. It wasn't like grit or guts or spunk or dependability; those things I sharpened through hard work. I felt lost because what mark had this persona I had created, Gracie Gold, really left on the skating world? Was all the artifice for nothing? If I couldn't be myself and I couldn't be a brilliant skater, then what the fuck was I even doing?

In the subjective world of figure skating, I sensed that my fuck-ups in that program were not just mistakes that had cost me a World Championships medal. The mistakes I made on April 2, 2016, would dog me for the rest of my skating career. They would subtly (and not) inform the commentary of the broadcasters who questioned my commitment and motivation and the judges who pegged me as someone who couldn't be counted on when the pressure was intense.

This would also end up being a pivotal year for my family, and not in a good way. Everyone was distracted by their own shit. No one had the patience to indulge my pain, to accept me where I was. "Grow up!" Carly told me. "You're being a baby!" Carly and my parents counseled perspective: "Do you know how many people would be thrilled to finish fourth at the world championships? We love you the same whether you got fourth or first."

It was as if they weren't seeing me at all. I was speaking the language of grief, and Carly and my parents were answering with platitudes.

I can remember a few distant acquaintances who said something to the effect of, *I hear you, Gracie. I see that something's wrong and that it probably has nothing to do with a botched toe loop or a popped triple Lutz.* But because they weren't members of my inner circle, their words failed to pierce my protective bubble.

What I think happened after Boston isn't that my fourth place finish impacted my life, but the other way around. My life bled into skating.

Competitive skating is three-pronged. There's the technical component, which I really enjoyed, and the creative side, which also filled me with joy. But to put the technical and creative parts together in a public performance requires being in a good headspace, and that was the part that I struggled with. I would make myself nervous and apply so much pressure to be the next Michelle Kwan instead of wholly myself. I compared every event to the Olympics, and every time out I demanded the same level of performance that I had delivered in Sochi, whether I was at a small summer competition or the World Championships. I was continuously chasing the Olympic high I had experienced—and falling short. It was almost as if I couldn't empty my mind of all the clutter and plant myself in the here and now, and in that way I became the architect of my self-destruction.

As time went on, a pattern emerged. The more chaotic my world became away from the ice, the harder it was for me to ground myself on it. Like I said, it's possible that somebody recognized what was happening and reached out and I simply wasn't receptive.

What is clear in retrospect is that I really would have benefited from taking an extended break to regroup after the World Championships. It's not unusual for a skater to sit out an entire season to heal a stress fracture in her foot, but it would have been considered highly questionable for someone to miss a whole season to mentally recharge—and especially not in the middle of an Olympic cycle. There's this ingrained belief that if you stop skating for no good physical reason, you'll forever lose your spark or edge. Skating is so intense—your medium, the ice, is so unforgiving—that you simply cannot skip a week of training, much less an entire season.

It's rarely spoken of openly, but I'm convinced that the primary reason we are encouraged not to take much of a break—why it is driven into us that we'll have plenty of time to rest after we retire—is because people typically put on weight when they stop training and the extra pounds are seen as a major obstacle in returning to peak form. But since that would be saying the quiet part out loud, we are encouraged, however tacitly, to talk about how we can't dream of a day without skating in it because "we love it so much."

It's terrible to say, but I'd probably have been better off if I had done something to hurt myself intentionally—dropped a heavy weight on my foot or something—so I'd have had an acceptable reason to step away from skating, one that didn't raise any red flags. How wack is that?

At the very least, I should have kept skating just enough to maintain my connection to the ice and taken a break from competition. Whatever oomph I lost on my jumps would have been more than made up for by the relief of escaping the hamster wheel. And speaking of the hamster wheel, I came across a random tweet once that hit me with the force of a commandment sent from on high: "The hamster wheel keeps spinning but the hamster is dead."

Looking back, I wish I had spoken up and said, *I should not be competing.* I advocated for a break, but not nearly forcefully enough. Nobody listened, or if they did, nothing came of it and eventually my depression was testing everybody's patience. People became exasperated with me when my blues didn't clear up like bacterial infections after a cycle of antibiotics. I was taken seriously for about a month or two, and then people's reactions were pretty much that it was time for me to "grow up" and "get over it."

My mistake was to pose my leave-taking as a question. It

should have been a declaration: *I'm taking this season off.* But if I had said that, it would have been interpreted as *She's giving up. Not stepping away because she needed a mental health break, but giving up because she was soft and weak, a baby who didn't have the competitive edge to leave a real mark on the sport.*

Olympic sports don't operate on a one-year calendar. Rather, it's a four-year cycle, and once you're into it as far as I was in 2016, it's full speed ahead. You hold it together until the end of a cycle, and then your issues can be addressed.

So, I kept going. I compartmentalized my feelings, stuffing my shame into one zippered pocket and my embarrassment into another. But that fourth-place finish was like a stench that I could not shake off. At the ice shows that I took part in, I'd be reminded during introductions and also at media availabilities that I was one of the skaters in the production that had failed to medal in Boston. I could not escape the shame of it. And so, like any untreated wound, that World Championships performance festered until it became an abscess on my psyche.

9

ARCHITECT OF MY OWN DESTRUCTION

The human brain was not engineered for what a skater is trying to accomplish. As soon as we start a spin on the ice, the motion sensors in the inner ear's semicircular canal are activated. An electrical signal is transmitted to the brain to alert it to the motion. Because of inertia, the sensors continue to register a false sensation of movement even after we stop, which is why the world still feels like it's spinning even though we're standing still.

I think of this concept every time I drive over a bump and the coffee in my Styrofoam cup continues to slosh around after the road evens out. Over the years, skaters' brains adapt to spinning by muffling that sloshing feeling in our heads after we've stopped.

If only I could equally train my brain not to short-circuit when I get angry. Instead, I react with one of two extremes: I shut down completely, like a turtle retreating into its shell, or I have a nuclear meltdown that eviscerates whoever's in my path. The safer and more secure I feel being vulnerable around you, the greater your chances of ending up downwind of my radioactive fallout.

Sorry in advance. I'm just stating the facts. To know the real me is to be occasionally savaged by me. It explains why my mom is a frequent target of my tantrums. My coaches and my boyfriend, too. I actually scream a lot less as an adult than I did as a child. When I shared that with my boyfriend, his response was that he's glad he didn't know me then.

A good rule of thumb: If I'm quiet or stoic around you, that's when you should be offended. It means I don't trust you with my big feelings. Take Frank, whose complaints about my bitchiness honestly surprised me because I rarely showed much emotion around him. We were never close enough for him to trip my temper. I might be hurt by something he said, but my plastic Barbie face wasn't easily dislodged by him.

I don't remember the first time I huffed and puffed and blew Frank's mind, but I can pinpoint when my behavior around him deteriorated. It was after Carly retired following her participation in the 2016 nationals. Because she knew me better than anyone else, she could defuse my anger or frustration with a single word or a glance or one arm around my shoulder. She was my emotional regulator, and when she no longer was around, I became increasingly unhinged. After she retired is when I began with some regularity turning tissue boxes, CD covers, and skating guards into projectiles, which surprised and unnerved Frank. Of course it did. He was so proper and poised. He didn't have the temperament or patience to manage unmasked Barbie. After he invariably failed to calm me down, he'd sigh and wearily say, "Time for the medics." It was a line played for laughs, but I failed to find the humor in it.

After she retired from skating, Carly enrolled in college. It hit me hard seeing her transitioning to the world beyond skating. I was happy and excited for her, but at the same time Carly's new life cast my own failure to thrive in a harsher light. I missed my emotional support buddy terribly. It was time to let her go, but I didn't want to.

She was off developing new friends and interests while I felt more stuck in the sport than ever. I had signed endorsement deals with companies that expected to cash in on my high profile and success at the 2018 Winter Games. I had begun filming Olympic promos and posing for magazine covers for Pyeongchang. Moving on was not an option for me.

I resented the freedom that Carly had. She didn't have to rise early in the morning to get to the rink. She didn't have to watch her weight to facilitate her jumps. And soon she had her first real boyfriend. Again, I was thrilled for her, but it was also unsettling because for the first time she had someone in her life more important in some ways than me. We had always been quick to introduce our BFFs by saying, "This person is my best friend—well, next to my sister," but now Carly really did have someone who could be there for her romantically, emotionally, academically . . . I felt not exactly replaced but sort of abandoned.

I was suffering from a phantom twin. Carly was gone most of the time, but I still felt so attached to her.

I became more distracted, more difficult to be around. I know Carly sometimes felt as if she were invisible when we were on the ice, but after she was gone her absence was palpable. Her anxiety about promptness and preparedness had kept me in check in ways I didn't fully appreciate until she was no longer there. I knew being late would send Carly off the rails, so even though I wasn't a morning person, I made sure to get up and out of the house so that we'd make it to the rink on time. It was difficult for me to manage my time and schedule without her, because between Carly and my mom I had never had to fend for myself.

I've always had trouble rising early. I'm an insomniac and a night owl, and have been pretty much since day one, but as spring turned to summer, I didn't even make an effort. I started sleeping the mornings away and arriving at the rink well into the afternoon. The first of my agoraphobic behaviors surfaced around this time. Instead of running outside in nature, which science suggests is serotonin for the soul, I limited my running to indoors on the treadmill. I wouldn't recognize how important being outdoors and communing with the natural world was until I entered therapy later and swimming, volleyball, hikes, and equine therapy became integral parts of my treatment.

The only aspect of my normal routine that I adhered to religiously was my diet. It was the last form of control that I had. On my "good" days, I managed to consume less than five hundred calories a day—three apples or three tomatoes plus coffee. Eating supplanted skating as the activity around which my days revolved. I was trapped in a terrible cycle in which I'd experience anxiety about appearing in a show or making a sponsor appearance or even taking a vacation because I was afraid of getting fat if I deviated at all from my rigid routine.

Whenever I felt overwhelmed by events, I leaned in to the light-headedness, the gastrointestinal distress, and my constant shivering due to my body's lack of fat (not good if your office is a refrigerated arena)—all side effects of my dieting. I was soothed by those sensations. Just writing those words, I am aware of how delusional I sound. Hello. That's why it's called mental *illness*.

If I didn't appreciate how much Carly helped me on the ice, I totally took for granted how much better she made life off the ice, as a sounding board for Mom and as the virtual glue holding our tattered family together. From the days she began chauffeuring us five hours each way from Missouri to Illinois and back, Mom had been an indispensable, ever-present force in our lives. There would be no Grace Elizabeth and certainly no Gracie Gold (but also maybe no Outofshapeworthlessloser) without Denise Gold.

But now Carly was spreading her wings and Mom was adjusting, badly, to her emptying nest. Carly was rarely home, and I couldn't blame her. She was *finally* putting herself first. For years she had served as the support system for me and Mom. Now she was choosing to save herself.

With Carly testing her independence, Mom tightened her grip on me. She'd call my phone repeatedly while I was on the ice to check on me. I remember on more than one occasion having a program run-through ruined by a phone call that interrupted my music. It was always Mom, and she would be indignant. "I haven't heard from you since you left at eight-thirty," she'd say. I had to bite my tongue to keep from screaming, *Are you my mother or my parole officer?* Instead, I'd sigh: "It's only eleven, Mom. I've been gone two and a half hours."

On weekends, Carly and I would go out to lunch, and if we weren't back in an hour, Mom would text one or both of us to ask where we were. "I just drove by the restaurant where you said you were going and I didn't see your car," she'd say. It hadn't occurred to her that we might have parked on a side street. It didn't matter that we had given her no reason to worry about what we were up to. I mean, neither one of us even had a fake ID. What trouble did she think we were finding? She became more and more suspicious of us, as if she had convinced herself that we were up to no good. At one point she started rifling through our belongings. I have no idea what she was expecting to find. A candy bar wrapper, maybe? I can't speak for Carly, but Mom's constant monitoring of me affirmed the belief that I was ill-equipped to move through the world as an adult—and that belief became a powerful incentive for me to keep skating.

I wish that I could have confided in Frank about any of this. But his strength was as a skating coach, not a life coach. His resting face was stoic. His old-world formality was impenetrable. Besides which, Frank adored my mom. For me in any way to taint his opinion of her struck me as selfish and downright shitty. She already had a terrible husband. I didn't need to make her feel worse.

Only recently did it dawn on me that Frank's emotional distance with me was probably *his* coping mechanism. Years before I came along, Frank had worked with another talented and temperamental singles skater. His name was Christopher Bowman, and Frank thought he was absolutely Olympic-champion material. He wasn't wrong. Christopher's nickname was "Bowman the Showman" for a reason. He had a big personality—and a bigger drug addiction. His first stint in recovery came as a teenager, before he won the first of his two World Championship medals in 1989.

Like me, he was a two-time U.S. champion. Also like me, he struggled with his weight. There's a famous story, passed down through the generations like an oral tradition, that Frank sat Christopher down once to impress upon him the importance of fueling his body like it was a Ferrari and not a Ford Escort, only to find out Christopher went out and bought three boxes of doughnuts and hid them under his bed. His mother found them and informed Frank, who insisted that she bring the doughnuts to the rink. Frank made Christopher eat every last one. And then, with a powdered sugar soul patch on his chin, he was ordered by Frank to do spins on the ice until he vomited.

It sounds harsh, I know, but by then Frank was out of answers. Their partnership started when Christopher was five years old and endured for almost twenty years, during which Frank developed a deep affection for him. Which made Frank all the more frustrated when he realized he was helpless to stop Christopher's self-destructive behavior. Frank eventually cut off contact with him as a tough-love measure, and they had no communication at all in the months leading up to Christopher's death from an accidental drug overdose in 2008. He was forty years old.

In an interview with *Time* magazine after Christopher's death, Frank said that he recognized two things could be true at once: He could love his skaters and hate some of their behaviors. He has been open over the years about the guilt that he has carried for having failed Christopher. I can understand, in that context, why Frank kept an emotional distance from me. He couldn't risk the heartache of getting sucked into another skater's emotional disturbances.

Frank wasn't stupid. He had an inkling that my diet was problematic before I brought up my weight with reporters in the fall. What was his first clue? My lethargy? My mood swings? My conspicuous consumption of energy drinks and coffee but not a single morsel of food during my seven hours at the rink? Actually, it was the old-fashioned lemon pound cake with cream cheese frosting that I made for him at the height of my *Cake Boss* phase.

Frank enjoyed every last bite, but it was so obscenely rich, he joked, it weighed almost as much as I did. For Frank, that cake was his lightbulb moment. My lavish baking did not square with my lean physique. Something was off. I might as well have brought him a box of doughnuts, so much did my gift transport Frank back to his days coaching Bowman. He attempted to open the line of communication several times: *"What can I do to help you? Is there anything you want to talk to me about? If there's some problem, let's get it out in the open.*" He expressed his concern in many ways, but he always got the same answer: "*Nothing's wrong.*"

I had worked so hard to be the perfect ice princess in front of Frank, it was hard for me to drop the mask around him. I get that I'm contradicting myself here. It's partly due to my not wanting him to hear anything negative about my mom that would possibly tarnish his high regard for her. But I also didn't know where to begin. We never had a super-close personal relationship, so it seemed wild to answer his question about what was wrong with something like "I think my parents are unhinged and I'm dissociating from reality."

There probably was a part of me that was hoping that in his wisdom he would divine what was wrong and help me fix it without my having to spell it out. At that point, I wasn't equipped to articulate what I needed from Frank. Our relationship was doomed from the start when I presented myself as the skater I believed he wanted me to be, hiding my ugly parts because I didn't think he'd want to work with me if he knew exactly what he would be dealing with. Because I wasn't honest with Frank, I never really gave him a chance to help me. I can't blame him for not knowing whether I needed help or was just one of the many spoiled brats he'd come across over the course of his half century in coaching. I'm not going to beat myself up for not having been more open, since I was on a probationary period of two weeks when we began working together. With terms like those, I knew I was skating on thin ice.

That's why, when Frank asked if anything was wrong, it was so much easier to say *I'm fine. Just out of shape.* To his credit, Frank connected me with a sports psychologist, Ken Ravizza, whose work with the Chicago Cubs was credited with helping them win the 2016 World Series title. I made some headway with Ken, but he suggested that I would be better served by clinical therapy.

The person Ken funneled me to I don't recall seeing more than once or twice. I didn't mind talking with Ken. His background in sports performance allowed me to skirt my family issues, which I was loath to discuss. I did not want a clinical psychologist poking at the hornets in our nest.

In the skating world, people were operating without much background or context, so there was no way they could identify what was wrong, much less help me. So I took matters into my own hands. I self-medicated with overexercise and undereating.

In August 2016, after Carly and I turned twenty-one, I added vodka, but sparingly at first. The upside of growing up in such a strict and conservative household is that even at my worst I never considered binge drinking. (Also, if I'm honest, it's a lot of calories.) The only time I drank liquor before I was twenty-one was at international competitions after I turned eighteen. To this day, I've never had a drink on an airplane and only once at an airport. I can't imagine my mortification if a young fan were to see me with an alcoholic beverage in my hand. Never mind that I am, as I write this, a grown adult of twenty-seven. It seems to me that children of alcoholics typically go one of two ways: either they replicate the drinking or they abstain from alcohol altogether. I fall more into the second category, though I'm not a teetotaler. I do my best to drink responsibly.

My experience is that most skaters party pretty hard. Which should surprise no one. In a sport that is so stifling and so rigid, why wouldn't skaters let loose when their events are over or at the end of the season? Recreational drugs are less prevalent. I have one or two friends that smoke the devil's lettuce—er, weed—on occasion to relax and unwind, but that's about the extent of it.

By the end of 2016, my *Firebird* program from nationals was the "high" I craved. If I could skate like that again, all the bad stuff weighing me down would evaporate. I almost convinced myself that the difference between broken and back was not unbridgeable. I wanted to believe that I wasn't too far gone. But the evidence to suggest otherwise was mounting fast.

10

"MY WORK IS DONE HERE"

People in figure skating can be so cavalier about how they talk about you. Coaches criticize your weight on a regular basis. Judges comment on your choice of dinner entrées or the clothes you're wearing in public. Journalists and television commentators shape their opinions of you around the story that they want to tell. And even the fans feel free to render judgment on your costume or your hairstyle or your sexuality or the authenticity of your smile. It takes great self-awareness to not fall into the trap of scrutinizing yourself with the same casual disdain as others do.

I recently found a clip on YouTube of my long program from Skate America in 2016. Held in suburban Chicago, the competition was utterly forgettable. The only aspect of it that was more cringeworthy than my performance—I fell on a triple loop and a triple Salchow, downgraded a couple of other triples, and nearly collided with the boards—was the commentary by the NBC team of Terry Gannon, Tara Lipinski, and Johnny Weir. Jesus fucking Christ! They went so far beyond breaking down my technical errors, it was as if they were channeling the radio talk show host

Dr. Laura Schlessinger, the high priestess of personal responsibility.

Their appraisal begins before my music to *Daphnis et Chloé* does. As I receive final instructions from Frank—"Fight . . . Take your time and be tough"—Terry remarks that it almost seems as if I'm seeking "confirmation, affirmation, if you will." Really? It sounded more to me like standard pabulum. Tara jumps in and says that I didn't seem resolute enough when I parroted back his words. "There's no determination behind it. There's no hunger. No anger," she says. Hungry? I was literally starving. I'm just saying.

One minute and forty-two seconds into my program, shortly after I end up on the ice after a failed triple loop, Tara says, "It's frustrating to watch. I'm going to make a bold statement and say that Gracie technically is way better than Ashley Wagner. So why she doesn't have the confidence to back it up, I don't know. I had to work very hard to be good technically. I didn't have the confidence all the time. But Gracie should just have it. She's that good."

Talk about backhanded compliments! If I may interject with a critique of my own: Tara was fifteen and built like a child when she won the ladies' Olympic gold medal at the 1998 Olympics. She had won the world championships the year before, but her rise was fairly meteoric, and she had the good fortune to be largely shielded from the kind of scrutiny she brings to her broadcasting work because she competed in the era of Michelle Kwan, who bore the burden of expectations as the face of U.S. ladies' figure skating at the time. With all due respect to Tara, how could she possibly understand what it's like to be twenty-one years old, as I was at this competition, with years of accumulated scar tissue from past disappointments and failures, knowing that if I wasn't perfect I was going to severely let down the world of figure skating yet again?

But I digress.

As I spin and step and jump apace, Terry responds to Tara's statement: "Don't you think she knows that, though, and it's why she went into quote-unquote a summer worlds depression?"

"I think so," Tara replies, "but it's time to snap out of it. It's been a while and either you're going to start to skate or not."

She's not done. A few seconds later, she says, "Beyond the technical mistakes, it's the look on her face. She just doesn't look like she wants to be out there."

Johnny pipes up. "It's hard to find that spark after you've had a lot of disappointing performances," he says. "But you've got to shake it off."

Snap out of it? Shake it off? You'd have thought I was on the rebound from a bad high school breakup or something. Okay, so they didn't know half of what was going on in my life during this time. Still, to say that I needed to "snap out of it" or "shake it off" was really overstepping their bounds. And here's the thing. A lot of viewers likely formed negative perceptions of me based on their commentary.

I know that if I had been watching, I probably would have thought, *Jesus, why should I root for this lazy, entitled bitch?* Which is truly unfortunate, since what people were really seeing was someone in the throes of a mental health crisis. Trust me, I wish I could shed depression and anxiety with a snap of my fingers or a shake of my booty. The commentary is so invalidating and so insensitive, let it stand as a teaching moment.

Since none of us really know what other people are going through, how about we stick to criticizing the performance, not the performer?

But no. After my music stops, Tara keeps going. "So many mistakes," she says. "I think she just has to go home and really dig deep and find that competitor. Because it's never going to work out for her if she doesn't learn how to attack."

Johnny says, "She needs to find Gracie Gold," and adds, "She needs to be herself on the ice and not portray the ice princess that she may not be."

Yes! This! Picking up Johnny's thread, Terry asks, "The great question is, and it goes beyond the ice, how do you find Gracie Gold?"

That was actually a great question. At that point, I had no answer. And neither did Frank. While we were in the kiss-and-cry area waiting for my scores, he said, without turning to look at me, "You looked tired." I responded, "There's a reason there aren't fat skaters."

Johnny and Tara didn't pick up on that exchange or chose not to comment on it, which is too bad. A discussion about the stresses of going through puberty in a light-body sport would have been enlightening to the audience—and relevant to the question that Terry had asked. Finding Gracie Gold was becoming more difficult as I was physically shrinking.

When I met with reporters after hearing my scores, an awkward exchange ensued. Asked to explain my error-laden performance and my disastrous fifth-place finish, I said, "We just need to adjust my physical shape and mental shape to see if the program can be salvaged."

I proceeded to use the word "overweight" to describe myself. I was under 120 pounds at the time, which a reporter pointedly noted.

"You are not overweight," she said. "You're slim."

My interview created a stir because I had said the verboten word out loud. Up until this point, nobody in skating had publicly addressed the elephant in the sport: the obsession with a certain type of thinness, an athletic leanness (an oxymoron, to be sure; it's the skating version of jumbo shrimp). It's interesting to me that people can express shock about disordered eating and body dysmorphia in a sport that requires you to carefully weigh yourself, your words, and your every interaction every day for years on end. You're skating in front of thousands of people in a small dress, and it's not just what you do that counts but how you look while you're doing it. The whole sport is based on random people judging you, so can we not simply acknowledge that under these conditions, being a top performer and dealing with a mental health crisis are not mutually exclusive?

As a light-body sport, figure skating pretty much requires all its athletes to constantly explore how far they can push themselves to fly without falling, not just on their skates but in their diets, their conditioning—everything. Whether it's a triple Axel or a double-digit weight loss, it's possible to extend yourself too far and not realize it until it's too late.

The rest of my 2016–17 season was a dumpster fire. Was I training every day? Yes. Was I executing my programs in practice every day? Sort of. I'd pop triples, ad-lib whole sections, and complete the program in a way that was unrecognizable to Frank. When he'd call me out on it, I'd challenge him. I'd say, "Well, I didn't stop."

Frank really hated working with me by then. And I really hated being me. So, contrary to what he thought, we were on the same page. I was focused on being thin, which meant exercising constantly. Strike that. "Focused" isn't the right word. I was committed to being thin. I wasn't focused on anything. I can't even tell you what I was thinking about. I was in this pea-soup fog and I couldn't find my way out of it. I didn't understand what was happening in my brain and what was happening to my family. I was completely detached, in a snow globe that I didn't know how to get out of. I challenged myself to marathon fasting periods and pushed the envelope. My personal best was forty-eight hours of subsisting only on coffee (while working out for five to seven hours a day). My body composition was easier to address than my family's deterioration.

My mom's drinking peaked in 2016, as far as I know. Naturally, I drew a straight line between my fourth-place finish at worlds and her increasing alcohol use. She had one daughter who had flown the coop, another daughter who was clearly spiraling, and an unfaithful husband in another state. If she wanted to have a beer or two to relax, who was I to argue?

If she was mixing sleeping aids and alcohol, well, as an insomniac, I could relate to her struggles. I noted the empty beer bottles under her bed and just put a pin in that observation. It was something we could deal with later. Eventually, though, there could be no ignoring the alcohol-fueled rages that Mom wouldn't remember the next morning.

My recollections of this time are of my intense but kind mother turning into a bad-tempered tyrant who threw objects like an empty laundry basket or cellphone across the room, bellowed insults, and was generally terrifying to be around. I knew her to be a screamer when provoked, but this explosive temper was something new. I wanted to ask, *Who are you and what did you do with caring, self-disciplined Denise?*

My mom's drinking is something we've never discussed, not even when I was in recovery. In typical Gold family fashion, it's one of those things that we've chosen not to comment on because to acknowledge it would lead to uncomfortable conversations. When Mom was blackout drunk, I'd be furious with her. But only for a moment. Then my anger would morph into guilt, because how could I be upset at the one parent who had sacrificed her life for me and Carly? My relationship with my mom could be summed up in two sentences: *I am very angry at you. But I don't want to make you upset.* To hear her talk, she was the child of shitty parents, now married to a shitty man. I had trouble staying mad at her or judging her because I could hardly handle my own issues. And if I ever found myself in her place, I'd probably want to be drunk most of the time, too.

One terrible night that I'll never forget, I arrived home from skating practice to find Mom in the kitchen of our open-concept house. As soon as I walked in the door, she began peppering me with random questions: "*What are your goals for the next competition? Are you training to the max?*"

What Carly and I had learned to do in these situations was give Mom enough of an answer to calm her down. But on this night, out of either fatigue or frustration, I took her bait. As I recall, I said something like "Are we really going to have this conversation when you're wasted?"

That did it. Mom tearfully regurgitated past hurts and injustices. She screamed at me. Carly was home, and Mom screamed at her. Carly got upset and stormed upstairs, and I followed her. We both were stopped dead in our tracks by a crashing sound. Mom had fallen and she was sprawled on the floor, surrounded by shards from a broken beer bottle. Things were said that night that opened my eyes to how bad things were in our family. The Good Ship Gold was taking on water fast, and if I couldn't bail us out with my skating, we were all going to sink.

I don't want to go too deep into the particulars because this part of my story is really Dad's to tell, but he has struggled for a long time with a prescription pill addiction. Unbeknownst to me or Carly, he had been disciplined by the state of Massachusetts for stealing medicine from a hospital in Boston for his personal use months before we were born.

In 2016, after another relapse, he was put on probation for misappropriating prescription drugs for personal use from a hospital in Illinois and subjected to mandatory drug screening. Dad failed to show for a December test, asked a handful of colleagues if he could borrow their urine, then submitted a clean sample the next day. His license would be suspended in February 2017, preventing him from practicing medicine for at least a year, but because he wasn't immediately forthright with my mom about what was going on, we'd continue on for a few months not knowing that the family's main source of income—Dad's salary—had dried up.

Carly was privy to more of what was going on than I was, which pissed me off. It infuriated me to know that I had been deliberately kept in the dark again. My whole life I was encased in this emotional Bubble Wrap when it came to family drama or strife. I could be screamed at about skating or my weight, but anything related to the outside world or my own family was strictly off-limits. Carly, meanwhile, was told pretty much everything and then instructed not to breathe a word to me. Carly had to carry the weight of the family's secrets. That was her cross to bear. Mine was being the family's hothouse flower, too precious or fragile to thrive outside the rink.

Mom and Dad were always full of reassurances. When I'd suspect that something was wrong and say something, they'd tell me, "You take care of the skating, and let us handle everything else." I was being shielded from the really ugly stuff so that it wouldn't negatively impact my skating, which was infantilizing. Did they think I couldn't handle the truth? It made me feel less like a family member than a show pony. *Gotta keep Gracie out of the loop so she can continue twirling across the ice with the greatest of ease . . .*

Skating got harder. My results got worse. Looking back, I can see that the problem was obvious: I was on high alert all the time from weathering the invisible aftershocks—or were they preshocks?—of our family's seismic upheaval.

The morning after the broken-beer-bottle night, Mom, Frank, and I left for a competition in Croatia. It was my last event before the 2017 nationals and I had absolutely no business being there. I didn't want to go. I had zero confidence in my ability to land a clean double Axel. I voiced my objections but was overruled by Frank and U.S. Figure Skating officials. I didn't fight it. By this point I was barely present in my own life. I was in no shape to make any podiums—or decisions.

Predictably, I earned my lowest international scores since 2012. Mom was so alarmed, she shifted into DEFCON 1. When we got back to Los Angeles, she met with Frank to discuss what could be done to salvage my season. It wasn't out of the ordinary for Mom and Frank to talk, though Frank would say years later that he had grown increasingly uncomfortable with their conversations during this period because Mom seemed to him to be under the influence of *something,* on occasion even slurring her words.

If Frank had any inkling that there might be a connection between my mom's behavior and my skating, he never brought it up. We were both well trained in maintaining skating's glossy veneer. *Nothing to see here. Move along.*

The offshoot of Mom's talk with Frank was that I should return to Alex in Chicago for a few weeks. He knew me as well as anyone. Maybe he could say or change something about my technique that would snap (there's that word again) my skating back into place. That we actually believed there might be a quick fix shows how deluded we all were. Frank was out of ideas, so he gave us his blessing. Maybe hearing a different voice would be helpful, he said.

I had misgivings about returning to Alex. There was a whiff of desperation to the move. It made me come across as vulnerable, which I obviously was. I just didn't need my rivals to know, lest they gain confidence at my expense.

Also, my attachment to Alex, seen with the benefit of distance, screamed "Stockholm syndrome." It wasn't exactly a healthy dynamic. But off to Chicago I went. By this point, I didn't have anything to lose, except for possibly more weight.

The sessions in Chicago went okay. Ahead of the nationals in Kansas City, Missouri, Frank told reporters that Alex's intercession appeared to have had a positive impact. Like Frank, I put on a brave face. I said I had forgiven myself for failing at the 2016 World Championships. (I lied. I still haven't gotten over it; it's possible I never will.) I was doing my best to channel the Halsey song lyrics that I had posted to my Instagram and Twitter pages before a successful stretch two years prior: "I'm meaner than my demons. I'm bigger than these bones."

Did I really think I could fake it until I could retake the national title? Not really. But as my mom had drilled into me when I was still a beginner, the show must go on. "I'm feeling so much better," I said. "I'm kind of falling back in love with the sport and with my programs and, most importantly, with myself."

Translation: *I lost five more pounds. My skating is shit, but it doesn't matter because I feel thin and pretty and proud of my small body, which I've worked so hard to shrink.*

Not surprisingly, I bombed. I was fifth after the short program, then went out and cleanly executed only two of my jumping passes in the free skate. I had to go back and watch a YouTube clip of my performance because I had no memory of the program. To be honest, all of 2016 is a blur. The only explanation I can offer is that I was stewing in so much stress, I was operating in a fugue state.

My friend Johnny Weir, in what I can objectively describe as scolding, said, "At this point it's time to grow up and skate." Ohkay. The presumption persisted that my skating went off the rails because I was immature or indifferent or insubordinate. It's the same way that Nicole Bobek, who won her only national title the year I was born, was spoken of, as was Tonya Harding before her. What the three of us had in common besides our blondness and our badassery was that we ate shit for so-called character flaws that one could argue were actually trauma responses to our environments.

Granted, my aesthetic didn't match Tonya's or Nicole's. No trailer parks or chain-smoking mothers in my youth. To the contrary, from the outside my life looked like a fairy tale, which probably confused people even more.

I finished ninth in the long program and sixth overall, which meant I failed to qualify for the World Championships. My absence from the Finland–bound U.S. team was a significant setback, because that event was the last major international test before the 2018 Olympics. To not be there would surely dim my stature in the eyes of the world's judges.

Waiting for my scores in the kiss-and-cry area in Kansas City, I remember I was seething. Frank was seated next to me, holding my Team USA jacket, water bottle, and cellphone. He asked me if I wanted any water, and I hissed at him, "No, I don't want any fucking water!"

I remember none of this. I had to reach out to others to piece together what happened because I was so checked out. I wasn't just done with skating. I had pretty much given up on life.

My publicist at the time met us backstage. She asked me if I wanted to review what I was going to say to the group of reporters waiting for me. She reminded me that I didn't want to say something in the heat of the moment that I'd later regret. Frank, concerned as ever with propriety, asked, "Would you like me to take this jacket or do you want to wear it?" I said something in the heat of the moment that wasn't nice. I snarled that he could throw my jacket in the trash for all I cared. It's funny, because I remember being lifeless save for a breath of sarcasm, but Frank's recollection is that I was spitting mad.

I walked away, leaving Frank standing there holding my belongings. Frank is a proud man, and after everything he had done for my skating, he didn't think he deserved to be treated like trash. His patience had run out. He would later describe me in that moment as "vicious" and "a monster." (I would have chosen "zombie," but whatever.) He walked to a garbage can situated between the group of reporters and the arena exit and, as the reporters craned their necks in his direction, he dumped my jacket in the trash can. "My work is done here," he said. "Good luck with your interview with Gracie."

Later, I dug my jacket out with as much dignity as I could muster.

Frank officially dumped me in a statement that he shared with IceNetwork.com. He said he couldn't envision us continuing to work together. He added, "When you spend a lot of time with somebody and give them all your energy and realize that it is now going nowhere, I think it is time for a change."

I'm not going to lie. It hurt to find out in the media that Frank and I were through. I released a statement, crafted by my management team, in which I attempted to strike a balance between gratitude and grievance: "I am surprised that Frank announced his decision before informing me. I continue to have the utmost respect for Frank Carroll and his legacy. He took me on during a very vulnerable time, and I am forever grateful for our work together."

I was being sincere. I was grateful that my two-week tryout with Frank lasted more than three years. At the same time, I wanted to convey that I was not washed up, even if Frank was insinuating as much by dumping me. I said that I intended to use the extra time not spent at the World Championships to prepare for the 2018 Olympic season.

The plan was to resume training full-time with Alex. My mom accompanied me to Chicago to help me find an apartment near the rink. But on the day that Alex and I had arranged to meet, he never showed. I dropped by the rink a few more times, but my enthusiasm waned with each day that Alex failed to appear. After two weeks, I accepted that Alex wasn't going to be my knight in shining steel blades.

My relationships with Mom and Carly were shaky, I had exhausted Frank's patience, and now Alex was ghosting me. It was devastating. My heart felt like it had been ripped from my chest and used in a dodgeball game.

If I had been thinking straight, I would have returned to Los Angeles, connected with the clinical therapist that Ken had found for me, and committed to the hard work of figuring out how I had wound up in such a dark place.

But I was not thinking straight. I had no thoughts at all save for this one. If my presence in skating is such a waste, what's the point of my taking up any space at all?

My options were limited, so I decided to move to Detroit to work again with Marina and Oleg, who had taken me in after I left Alex the first time. I told myself that all I needed was a change in scenery. *Change your address, change your life.* Who was I kidding? I didn't move to Detroit to rekindle my gold medal hopes. I went there for the same reason the family dog wanders off to some secluded spot to die. I wanted to spare my loved ones from my sad demise. Living on my own for the first time in my life, my downward spiral accelerated. On my own, I could no longer bear the weight of a terrible secret that I had been carrying.

11

INNOCENCE LOST

Something happened around this time that severely compromised my ability to "snap out of it" and "grow up and skate." Something that left me so traumatized that I was in complete survivor mode for much of the next year. Something that scarred me in ways I'm still processing.

The story of my trauma starts with a photograph. Looking at it now, I can see that I've let down both my guard and my hair, which has been liberated from its high bun and is framing my smiling face. How I wish I could warn that beaming twenty-one-year-old that not every person has her best interests at heart. Because shortly after the camera lens captured that photograph, my virginity was forcibly taken.

I knew my rapist because his and Carly's social circles overlapped. Our paths had crossed at a few international skating events over the years. I would eventually report him to U.S. Figure Skating and the U.S. Center for SafeSport, the organization that began operations in 2017 to investigate abuse in sports. But almost five years after I filed my complaint, my rapist was still competing with his reputation intact.

I think about my time line whenever I hear people wonder aloud why more survivors don't report their sexual assaults. Almost five years is more than an entire Olympic cycle. That's a long time to wait for closure for an event that continues to haunt me. And I'm not the only one. From what I've gathered, there might be multiple women who were assaulted by my rapist, including one survivor who was a minor at the time.

In the lead-up to the assault, my step was as light as it had been in a long time. It had been a godforsaken stretch, but I'd been skating better and was hopeful that a party at the end of an upcoming event would offer an escape from the stresses and strains I had been under.

After-parties are a fixture in skating, the gala after the final skating gala, if you will—an opportunity to let loose after days, weeks, and months of being tightly wound. I can remember a particularly memorable party after the Four Continents competition in Japan. One national team—not ours—trashed the entire floor of a hotel. It wasn't entirely their fault; they had lots of help from skaters from other countries. I vaguely recall someone executing a handstand in the hallway and putting both heels through the drywall. Another skater tore off an Exit sign. Somehow, the door to one room was liberated from its hinges. And a bag of stuffed animals that had been collected on the ice was emptied, turning the entire floor into what looked like a plush-toy graveyard. The members of the national team that occupied the floor had to issue a formal apology to the hotel before they were able to check out.

Which is all to say I was not a prude. I knew that after-parties could get rowdy. But when about a half dozen of us ended up back in the fancy suite that Carly and I had scored at our hotel, I wasn't worried at all that things could get out of hand. I looked at this after-party as more of a gathering, raising a toast to getting through a difficult year, than a rager. Because of the spaciousness of our accommodations, we were the designated hostesses. The alcohol was flowing freely. I don't even remember who was pouring the vodka shots, but I do recall belting down several of them on an empty stomach. By the time the festivities broke up, I was incapacitated. I was not blackout drunk. I know that much because I have a devastating recall of what happened next.

Carly and her boyfriend disappeared into the bedroom, and I clumsily attempted to open the sleeper sofa in the sitting room. While I was fumbling with the metal frame, I realized I was not alone. My rapist was dawdling in the background. It was an open secret that he had a crush on me. People would kid me about it. He had been awkwardly circling me for months. We went on one date that was memorable for our lack of chemistry. He was never going to get far with me, not with pickup lines like "I've entered a kissing contest, can you help me win?"

Unbeknownst to me, my relationship status was a source of curiosity in the skating world. One coach constantly pumped Frank for information. Why was a beautiful girl like me not romantically linked with anybody? The subtext was clear: *What's wrong with her?* Frank's answer was always some variation of "She's completely devoted to skating right now."

He wasn't wrong. But it went deeper than that. I hadn't met anyone I liked or trusted enough to be vulnerable around. Which is a roundabout way of saying that my history of sexual exploration was nonexistent.

I remember registering my rapist's presence in the room and thinking, *Why is he still here? Party's over, bud.* But as long as he was there, I figured he might as well make himself useful. I asked if he could help me figure out how to pull out the mattress. At some point after we had unfolded the metal frame, he pinned me down and started kissing me and rubbing against me. I remember very clearly saying, "No. I don't want to do this. Please. Not now." I was probably too polite at first. And too quiet, because I didn't want to disturb Carly in the next room.

I wish I had disturbed Carly in the next room.

My rapist was considerably stronger than me. As he became more forceful, I remember very clearly saying, "No thank you. I'm good," as if he were asking me if I wanted a glass of water. My brain was operating on a three-second delay.

Ignoring my pleas, he forced himself inside me. Mercifully, it was over fast.

The trauma of being sexually assaulted distorts your memory and alters time. I woke up a few hours later and he was gone. In the absence of any proof that he had been there, I actually wondered if the assault had been a terrible nightmare—until I untangled myself from the bed covers and saw the blood on the sheet. I took a quick inventory of my body and noticed that I was aching in places where I had never been sore before.

When you are sexually assaulted after a night of drinking, your shame is bottomless. I ended up essentially gaslighting myself. The story I told myself is that it wouldn't have happened if only I had been sober. My intoxication became the laceration on my character that I threw salt on. I told myself that if I'd had my wits about me, if I'd stuck to drinking cranberry-and-sodas, my rape would not have happened. That was the story I repeated to myself. I was humiliated and desperate not to jeopardize my reputation—especially as the face of a sport that traffics in a virginal type of beauty—and so I stuffed every memory of what happened into the furthest recesses of my mind.

I didn't speak about it, not even to Carly, which created an emotional distance between us. It magnified my guilt, shame, and self-disgust not to be able to share this terrible thing that had happened to me with the person that I'm closest to in this world. Knowing that my rapist had a schoolboy crush on me mortified me. I wondered if I'd somehow sent him the wrong signals, which was ludicrous, since sexual assault is not an act rooted in love or affection. It is about asserting power and control.

I don't regard my rapist as a predator who stalked me. I see him as an opportunist, the lion who waited in the savanna and then pounced when the giraffe was half-dead. A rumor got back to me that sent my humiliation through the roof. I hope to hell it isn't true, but I heard that he and another skater were in a contest to see which one could have sex with more female national champions. If that's the case, the contest rules clearly didn't require gaining the women's permission first.

I could have stopped at the police station on my way out of town and filed a police report. But what would I have submitted as evidence? A deflowered virgin's bloody bedsheet? Because I had been drinking, I didn't believe that I'd have any credibility in the eyes of the authorities. Then there was the matter of that earlier date plus another time when my rapist and I had made out, all of which left me wondering if I had misled him somehow. Would those two earlier consensual interactions shade how my assault was judged by others? Would they cloud the facts of what happened in that hotel room?

My confidence that my case would stand up in court was zilch. Less than zero, actually.

This person who had a reputation as a class clown was anything but harmless. How could I warn others when anything I said would likely devolve into a he-said-she-said situation? Would people believe that he was so starved for affection that he forcibly took it from me? Or would I end up being victim-shamed as an unreliable slut?

I returned with Carly to Los Angeles and life went on as normal. Over the holidays, Dad flew out from Illinois to spend Christmas with his "girls." Mom was always in full elf mode and I don't remember this holiday being any different. One year she gathered driftwood from the beach, sanded and sealed each piece, and arranged them like branches to form a tree, then created ornaments out of seashells that she also retrieved during her ocean walks and hung them from the branches using yarn. Mom maximized her powers of creativity to make the holidays festive, which maybe explains why Dad waited until several weeks into the new year before telling Mom he had been suspended from his job due to the missed drug test.

Eventually, I would share my secret with Carly—and immediately regret doing so. She was racked with guilt because as she saw it, my rapist had gained access to me through his connection with her.

A month later, Carly threw a party and I was adamant: My rapist was not to be invited. He showed up anyway, and I spent the entire night doing my best to dodge him. At one point he trapped me in the laundry room, grabbed me, and shoved me up against the washer. I escaped, but not before bloodying my leg. His pursuit of me became so aggressive that others at the party noticed and confronted him: "For real, stop! It's not funny. You're being weird." None of the partygoers were aware of what had happened earlier, but my rapist was making *everyone* uncomfortable. Finally, one of the guys at the party had seen enough. He told him to get the fuck out.

The next morning, a group of us met for brunch, and my rapist had the nerve to show up. He was quickly shooed away by two of my dining companions, who could see that the sight of him was upsetting to me.

In 2017, the actor Sarah Polley, who endured a sexual assault in her teens, wrote an op-ed in *The New York Times*. She said there's no right way for sexual assault survivors to proceed. It felt as if she were speaking directly to me when she said, "In your own time, on your own terms, is a notion I cling to when it comes to talking about these experiences of powerlessness."

I took the first tentative steps toward reclaiming my power while I was in recovery. During a talk session, I mentioned the assault, and after I described what happened my therapist encouraged me to contact the proper authorities, not just for my own benefit but because my rapist was around other women at his rinks.

On her advice, I reached out to Mitch Moyer. I felt super weird telling him what had happened. I didn't feel close enough to him to be confiding something so personal, and I wasn't sure I could trust him. The conversation was extremely awkward, and I was shaking when I got off the phone. But it was a necessary discomfort because I wanted to protect other athletes from becoming my rapist's next victims.

I remember Mitch sounding sympathetic. I remember him saying, "I'm sorry that happened. Thank you for telling me. You realize that I need to report this?"

The U.S. Center for SafeSport, an organization authorized by Congress and created with the goal of identifying and punishing people in Olympic sports guilty of sexual, emotional, and physical abuse, was just getting up and running. Mitch said he reported my incident, as he was required to do. I've been told that the police whose jurisdiction includes the rink where my rapist was training at the time were also alerted, but nothing came of the information that was passed on to them. More than two years went by, and I heard nothing from Mitch about my case and not a peep from anybody at SafeSport.

My experience, it seemed, was being invalidated. But then, shortly before COVID-19 brought the world to a virtual halt, Mitch called me. It was late at night, and I almost didn't pick up the phone. He wanted me to know that someone from SafeSport would be calling me the next day. Inappropriate behavior in figure skating was back in the news. A figure skater who was born outside of the United States but was training in America had been implicated in a different case. It apparently brought new attention to my case. I would end up speaking to someone with SafeSport. The person entrusted with taking my information opened the conversation by saying that he and his wife were huge fans of mine. It was awkward, to say the least. *Oh, thank you. Now let me tell you how I was raped.*

I would have been far more comfortable speaking with a woman than with this older white gentleman who professed to be a big fan. But it wasn't up to me. In any event, that was the last I heard from anyone about my case.

I've since learned that there's been a change in case managers. But still no resolution. In the meantime, my rapist continued on with his career. Subsequently, my coaches reached out to U.S. Figure Skating and SafeSport to help me avoid my rapist on the competitive circuit without any prompting from me because that's what responsible and caring individuals in positions of authority do. They have their athletes' backs. They reminded the powers that be that there was—and still is—an open case in Safe-Sport against him, that it would be extremely uncomfortable for me to bump into him, and that if I did encounter him, I could make it extremely uncomfortable for everyone by blurting out in an interview something to the effect of, *Well, I was a little dis*tracted *at practice on account of my rapist being in the building.*

I've read that when someone experiences a crisis, one of two things happens: They don't recover. Or they do recover and are irrevocably changed by the act of pulling through. There is no third option. A person does not emerge from a crisis unchanged. I can absolutely see the truth in that. I survived the assault, but when I consider that photograph from before it happened, I barely recognize the trusting person staring back at me.

12

"IS THIS THE RIGHT TIME?"

Stripping and ice skating. They're among the few disciplines in the United States where women attract way more eyeballs and enjoy more earnings potential than men doing the same thing.

Makes sense if you think of it. I'm not so different from a pole dancer; we both traffic in the art of seduction.

It's interesting to me that if I stripped, I'd widely be dismissed as corrupted. But because figure skaters keep our tiny skating costumes on, we are held up as paragons of virtue. It's unfortunate, because if you look past our packaging we're selling the same thing: institutionalized sexism.

That's why it doesn't surprise me in the least that a handful of skaters I've known have graduated to the sex industry after their competitive days are over. I respect that they are being financially compensated—and, well, I hope—for being objectified, for perpetuating a female ideal that they once maintained at great physical and emotional cost for little, if any, monetary gain.

How many years did I spend hating my thighs because my muscled legs, however central to my success, did not conform to the version of femininity that equates figure skating with pretty girls in pleasing dresses with pipe-cleaner limbs?

A question I recently fielded from a teenage skater brought me up short. She asked, "Why isn't my natural face beautiful enough?" On the surface, she was asking why the thick show-girl makeup is necessary. But I understood the subtext: *Am I not pretty enough on my own to be a skater?* "You have a beautiful face," I assured her, "but it's a great question." I said I wished I had a great answer, "but I can't tell you when skating or society is going to change." In the meantime, I encouraged her to think of makeup differently—as something that's not covering her imper-fections but, rather, enhancing her features so they can be seen from the seats farthest from the ice.

Long hair in a bun is also a must—and the higher the bun the better. The days of 1976 Olympic champion Dorothy Hamill's short, bouncy wash-and-wear wedge cut are long gone. My hair fell down my back for most of my life. After my stay in recovery, I had it chopped shorter than shoulder-length. New me, new look. People in skating reacted with such horror, you would have thought I had tattooed my forehead.

Among the conservative WASPs who have ruled figure skating in America from its elitist beginnings, short hair on women is a dog-whistle feature associated with lesbians. Which is not ideal in a sport that sells its female stars as if we're starfish: beautiful to behold but asexual.

For all its sensual music and alluring costumes, skating is off-puttingly prudish. It's hypertraditional, almost toxic in its strait-laced, God-fearing palatability. In America, this model has not aged well. Despite the progressiveness of its participants, the sport still celebrates a retrograde suburban image of what ath-letes should be. Not for nothing, I've heard people high in the U.S. Figure Skating hierarchy refer to Asian Americans as "Orientals," as if they were rugs or chicken salad. That's sadly where the culture is at. It's stuck in the 1950s.

Unlike the stripper, who can shed her persona as soon as she steps off the stage, I have been commanded to wear my skating costumes off the ice. As if they are my second skin. Seriously. While the 2022 Winter Olympics in Beijing were going on, I was invited to be a guest on an Olympics highlights show hosted by the actor and comedian Kevin Hart. I was told to wear my glam skating dress.

The retired NFL star Michael Irvin also was a guest. Did he show up in his game-day tights? No. He did not. As I looked at him all comfy in his street clothes while I stood freezing in the 32-degree chill of the curling rink, my teeth chattering so loudly that it ruined a couple of takes, my mind flashed to all the police procedural drama series reruns that I had binge-watched while holed up in my Detroit apartment. Despite my depressive fog, it wasn't lost on me that the women officers always wore low-cut blouses to carry out their investigations while their male cohorts were dressed more conservatively and comfortably.

Even when the entertainment isn't about sex appeal, it's about sex appeal.

And it's not just skating. It's everything. The American lesbian activist and author Elana Dykewomon was spot-on when she said, and I'm paraphrasing here, that women spend almost every waking hour on guard—hyperalert to the vibes we are sending off and receiving, and hyperaware of the need to control our tempers, appetites, sexuality, feelings, and ambitions. And then people wonder why we often seem to be "hysterical."

The overwhelming assumption in skating is that every woman is straight and every man is gay. Not everywhere, but certainly in the United States, it is presumed—by those who would reductively categorize it as a "feminine" sport—that men who skate must not, cannot, be straight. I've seen judges and officials who talk a good game when it comes to tolerance award lower scores to skaters who aren't performatively masculine (see Johnny Weir's career).

Ahead of the Beijing Olympics, Nathan Chen sat for a podcast interview. He was asked if people wonder why he didn't choose hockey, since it is considered a more masculine sport than figure skating. Nathan gave an honest answer. He said that as a straight male "in a fairly LGBTQ-dominated sport," he is aware of that perception, which he described as "messed up in itself," and added, "We spend our whole lives trying to hone this craft, and to be just sort of belittled like that is not something that is generally taken lightly."

Two decades earlier, the HBO hit series *Sex and the City* had played for a punch line a similar sentiment. In a third-season episode, Carrie informed her friend Samantha that a guy she was interested in romantically was bisexual. "I could've told you that, sweetie," Samantha replied. "He took you ice skating, for God's sake."

I'm glad Nathan spoke his mind, though I also understand why he drew criticism from the LGBTQ+ community and the skating world. Nathan suggested that being considered gay was belittling, a comment that revealed how deeply homophobia still lives within people's minds. Later, he said he had fumbled an op-portunity to disabuse people of the notion that there are such things as masculine or feminine sport, and to illuminate the ways in which that erroneous perception fosters an environment "that makes it unsafe, stigmatizing, and even career-ending for ath-letes to come out."

Still, Nathan had touched on the generalized internalized ho-mophobia that still exists. As a woman in the sport, I was readily accepted by everyone, everywhere. Nathan's experience made me wonder: Would I have been seen as America's skating sweetheart if it was widely known that my romantic partners included men *and* women?

I haven't hidden my bisexuality. I didn't see the need to come out because I never considered myself closeted. My first serious girl-friend was a woman I'll call Ellen. She was outspoken and loudly herself, with a trigger-quick sense of humor. In an environment filled with pretenders, she definitely stood out. She was the first person to tell me that I gave off vibes that I liked women—though I suspected after watching Missy Peregrym and Kellan Lutz in the gymnastics movie *Stick It* when I was ten that I was equally attracted to men and women.

I was attracted to Ellen because she was everything that I was not. She was rough around the edges where I was polished to a shine, reckless where I was reserved. She lived her private life without weighing the public consequences, whereas I weighed the public consequences before living my private life. I was im-pressed that Ellen had a plethora of tattoos and no fucks to give about what anybody thought of her. She followed her own happi-ness, even when it led her to bad places. She had had several brushes with the authorities, I'm just saying. It was a relief to shed my perfectionism and go with the flow when we hung out.

She told me she had been a softball player with a college schol-arship in her sights until an injury ended her athletic career and led to an addiction to pain medication and the aforementioned run-ins with police. It wasn't as if her pattern of drug and alcohol abuse was the result of her being a party animal or ne'er-do-well. Her addiction came from a place of trauma, which resonated with me since my eyes were beginning to open to allow me to see people differently. Less judgmentally. The black-and-white world of my conservative midwestern childhood was disappearing, eclipsed by a diorama filled with grays. Not everyone who uses drugs is a "junkie." Not every girl with her tits out is a "slut." Not every unhoused person is a dangerous schizophrenic. I was waking up to the scars that pain and trauma can inflict on people and how it was nobody's business—certainly not mine—how people chose to heal.

Other friends in Los Angeles sensed that my rapport with Ellen was flirty. It opened me up to some good-natured teasing. I'm sure a few were dubious. There are people, I've discovered, who hear "bisexual" and think "confused." Their attitude is *Pick a team, already!* I dated a man who said he had misgivings about going out with a bisexual woman because the pool of people I could cheat on him with was twice as large. *Hmm, tell me you're insecure without telling me you're insecure.*

At some point, one of my IMG agents reached out to me. As I recall, she was uptight. A reporter was chasing down a lead that I was dating a woman, she said. "Okay," I replied. "Is that a problem?"

"Well, yes and no," she said. Her advice to me was that any "coming out" disclosure would have to be handled delicately. In a voice laced with concern, she asked, "Is this the right time?"

I found the question offensive. Had I fallen asleep and woken up in 1980? She explained that Rudy Galindo had benefited from staying in the closet. I wanted to believe that the culture had evolved since Rudy skated in the 1980s and '90s. I failed to see that my safety was at risk since I already had male stalkers, which suggested that heterosexuality could be a security concern. So what was the source of the unease? I quickly realized that what they were really worried about was public palatability. The irreparable damage it would do to my ability to make money for myself—and for them—if I didn't conform to the heterosexist ideal. I don't remember if I asked it outright, but I know I was thinking: *Are you asking me to lie? Or to beat around the bush* (no pun intended)?

I wasn't worried about being outed as bisexual. I was physically attracted to someone of the same sex. So what? If my relationship with Ellen was divulged, would it not at least send a positive message, affirming that there is room in skating for everybody? Either way, I failed to see why my romantic choices were anybody's business. I said the concern that the revelation of my bisexuality would invite bad press was messed up. I truly didn't think anybody would care.

My management team persisted. "What if people ask you about your sexual orientation?" Again, so what? Even as a child, I struggled with the idea that someone would hurt someone else or think less of them because of who they chose to love. I remember asking my mom what a hate crime was, and she gave the example of people who will perpetuate violence on LGBTQ+ people because they view those individuals' orientation as a crime against God. I was confused. Aren't all of us God's creations? Mom shrugged. All she could do was acknowledge the flawed logic.

I wouldn't have been the first LGBTQ+ woman in skating anyway. Around this time, the ice dancer Karina Manta came out as bisexual. She was the first openly queer female figure skater to compete for Team USA. Her skating partner, Joe Johnson, is gay, so they made history at Skate America as the first openly queer ice-dancing team.

Before Karina, there was the two-time Japanese Olympian Fumie Suguri, who waited until she retired to reveal her bisexuality in 2014. The United States singles skater Amber Glenn announced in 2020 that she identifies as bisexual and pansexual.

Then there's Kaitlyn Weaver, a U.S.-born two-time Olympic ice dancer for Canada, who came out as queer in 2021. She said she waited until after she was done skating because she was afraid that if the judges knew the truth about her, her scores would have been docked. Like a married couple in a TV series, ice dancers are expected to act like lovers no matter how they feel about each other when the cameras go dark.

The call ended with me saying that if I was asked about my sexuality, I would tell the truth, and whatever happened next, so be it. For whatever reason, nobody ever asked. My management team never brought up the subject again.

I was still in the casual friendship stage with Ellen when I started receiving inappropriate texts from an Olympic champion from Russia. He was nearly twenty years my senior, lived in the Los Angeles area, and was newly divorced. He'd randomly show up at the rink where we trained, pop off a few triples to show he still could, and leave. None of us were clear about why he showed up during our sessions. He made comments about my body, including one about my "big ass." Unsure what to do, I shared the messages with Ellen and eventually showed them to Frank, who went through the proper channels to have the skater banned from our rink. It blows my mind to consider that there are some in figure skating who might have found my attraction to Ellen more disturbing than this much older skater's preoccupation with my body.

My friendship with Ellen didn't deepen into something beyond that until after I moved to Detroit. We carried on this weird long-distance courtship, if you can call it that, for about six months. She provided camouflage for me at a time when I didn't want to be seen. My sister and mother considered Ellen a terrible influence and questioned her motives. They wondered if I wasn't unconsciously replicating in my connection with her all the drama of my family dynamics. I was equating chaos with excitement, they said, as a way to deal with stress.

What they failed to recognize was that everything that they scorned about Ellen was precisely what attracted me to her. Unlike anyone in my family or anyone in skating, Ellen modeled a way to live your life that wasn't plastic in any way. She lived by no one's rules—not her family's, not society's, and certainly not some sports federation's. She wasn't going through "a phase."

While we were together, Ellen applied for a job that would have been a step up in prestige and salary. She went through the interview process and was offered the job only to turn it down. I was flabbergasted. What was she thinking? The company had made it clear that she would have to dress differently—to hide her forearm tattoos under a long-sleeved blouse, for starters.

"Why would I want to work someplace that wanted me to change who I was fundamentally?" she said with a shrug.

I couldn't believe it. She was giving voice to a concept that doesn't fucking exist in skating. Being yourself at whatever cost was the most radical thing I'd heard in my life.

Who *am* I, anyway? The question is like a ball of yarn that I keep pawing at. During a 2022 trip home to Los Angeles, I attended an adult hockey league game with my mom. We were there to watch Carly, who was playing for a team named after a hard-seltzer beverage. She looked adorable in her lime jersey.

Carly spent so much time freezing her ass off in cold arenas cheering me on. Now it was my chance to return the favor, be her No. 1 fan. From the opening face-off, I yelled until I was hoarse: "Push, Carly, push!" And "Get him, Carly!"

Mom noted my enthusiasm. She mentioned something about the hockey lessons I had asked for all those years ago in Springfield, Missouri. She had to refresh my memory. I closed my eyes and imagined little Grace Elizabeth battling in the corners for loose pucks. I could totally picture it. I was such a tomboy. I bought my clothes, especially hoodies, in the boys' section, turned my nose up at makeup and jewelry, and was in-your-face aggressive. I would not have shied away from contact.

If I had played hockey, how would it have shaped my personality? My life? And if I hadn't been incentivized to become an ice princess, would my private and public selves have been more aligned? I can't discount the possibility that Outofshapeworthlessloser took root in the space between the two, like a weed growing through a crack in the cement.

13

FAILED ANOREXIC

The seven months that I spent in Detroit in 2017 are mostly lost to memory's dustbin. All I can offer from this period are pixelated images that, like shifting sands, have rearranged themselves over time. There's so much for which I have no recollection. Conversations, competitions, entire weeks were wiped from my brain by some sprinkler system activated when my brain caught fire.

In a journal entry I unearthed from around this time, I wrote:

You do nothing but worry.

You worry about your skating, your weight, your image, and what other people think of you.

You don't like this new you, but you aren't doing anything to change.

I was unable to move on or make any progress because I could not shift out of survival mode. It was like I was offline, out of it. I think the psychological term for it is "dissociating." Again, the best way I can describe it is the snow globe analogy. I could see the world beyond my bubble, but I couldn't access it. On occasion, people would tap on the glass to get my attention, but it was like there was a barrier between us that kept me from making myself heard or understood.

I was a ten-minute drive from the Canton rink used by my new coaches, Marina Zoueva and Oleg Epstein, but mentally I was a million miles away. Marina was known for her success with ice dancers and had worked the previous summer with Nathan Chen. Oleg had collaborated with Alex once upon a time, and I supposed I looked at him, in my desperation, as an Alex surrogate: someone who, by his mere presence, could choreograph me into being the skater I was in Chicago. Marina and Oleg are excellent coaches. They were not the reason I failed to thrive. For every day that I put in a bare minimum of two on-ice sessions and a gym workout upstairs at the rink, there'd be three or four where I struggled to find the energy to brush my teeth or hair.

I can remember thinking, *Why should I brush my hair when I'm not going anywhere? What's the point? Why should I take a shower when the sight of my body repulses me? Why bother?* I was slowly withdrawing from the world. Nobody was going to see me. I was caught in a vicious cycle. My depression made any kind of movement effortful, and the less active I was, the more depressed I became.

I put the skaters in Detroit who knew me only by reputation in a tough spot. They weren't familiar with my habits, so maybe they just thought I was eccentric. It's possible they didn't pay attention to me at all since they were preoccupied with their own pre-Olympic preparation. Looking at my demise through their eyes, I can understand why I could have been perceived as a drama queen or lost cause. I was very aware of how I must have come across to the outside world—as the same person Frank saw, someone richly blessed who had squandered her many gifts.

During this time, I continued to pose for Olympic-themed photo shoots and commercial spots as if nothing was amiss. *The show must go on!* I continued to meet with reporters and talk a good game about my training and preparation. All the attention only increased the anxiety I felt not to let everybody down, but in the short term, the photo shoots and interviews served a valuable purpose, forcing me to go to the rink when I might have otherwise stayed home. I'm sure Marina was worried about me. But nobody wanted to risk upsetting me by saying what they were really thinking. Skaters are trained to sell a performance no matter how badly it's going. So I can understand if everybody shrugged off my lethargy, assuming I'd pull out of my spiral in time to do my job in Pyeongchang.

I'll never forget an interaction I had on the ice during this time. This person had grown exasperated with my "act," as they described it. Under the guise of being helpful, and with a straight face, they delivered this pearl of wisdom: "Gracie, if you want to be happy, be happy." I hadn't thought it was possible to weigh north of 150 pounds and go unseen, but in that moment I truly felt invisible. What was I supposed to do with that advice? *Oh, thank you so much. Let me turn my frown upside down right now.*

There must have been days during this time when I didn't feel depressed and antisocial and unloved and unlovable. I've heard from people who were in Detroit then that I was fun at parties. Marina remembers me being a hard worker when I showed up. What stands out in my mind is how I just barely maintained appearances. The footprints I left each day were faint enough to raise some red flags but not enough to trigger a full intervention. I went out socially enough for people to register my existence. I could still summon the energy, once in a while, to be the life of the party. But mostly I fought a losing battle against apathy. I didn't feel right, but I couldn't pinpoint exactly what was wrong.

A voice in my head would be urging me to go to a SoulCycle class or spend an hour at the gym. In the past, that voice—my conscience, I suppose, or maybe my killer instinct—would be enough to spur me to do what needed to be done. But it was having no effect on me. I was like, *Meh.* I assumed I had a motivation problem, not a mental illness.

When I say I was in bad shape, this is what I mean: I chose not to carpool to practice because I didn't want to be accountable for showing up. I avoided going outside, so much so that I became borderline agoraphobic. I slept entire days away and then stared at the TV for seventy-two hours straight in an insomniac stupor. I binge-watched all eight seasons of *Dexter* because what is more on-brand for a depressive living a double life as an Olympic gold medal contender than watching a drama about a sociopathic serial killer? I watched *Game of Thrones* for the escapism. On days when I stepped away from the remote and made it to the rink for a session or media appearance, I first had to hole up in the bathroom until the waves of panic subsided.

As depression settled into my bones, my starvation diet gave way to binge eating. I went from consuming one apple or tomato a day to two delivery pizzas in one sitting. The comfort food was satisfying a bottomless anxiety, an unending shame that fed on itself.

I put on ten extra pounds, then twenty and thirty. Bingeing took over my life the way skating once had. Every aspect of my day revolved around it because of the secrecy required in acquiring and eating so much food. My self-loathing grew along with my waistline. *My God, I can't even succeed at starving myself,* I thought. I might as well have been walking around wearing a sandwich board that proclaimed FAILED ANOREXIC.

After consuming thousands of calories at a time, mostly in carbs, I'd purge them by activating my gag reflex, but over time I lacked the energy or motivation to do that. So on top of everything else, I became a failed bulimic. My weight climbed to 160, then north of 170. I was embarrassed to exist, ashamed to take up so much space in the world. I was by myself but not alone. Mean, judgmental, sarcastic Outofshapeworthlessloser was living rent-free in my head: *You're not messed up. You're fat and that's all on you. That's your fault. Nobody is force-feeding you. You lack discipline. You are disgusting. A joke. You look like a potato with arms. You're just wasting your life. If you just killed yourself, you never would have had this problem. You'd have zero problems.*

I'll say this for Outofshapeworthlessloser: She's awfully persuasive.

Nobody wants to look at their reflection and see Ms. Potato Head, so I covered every mirror in my apartment, only to discover later, somewhat fittingly, that people in the Victorian era did the same thing after someone died. I was still alive . . . but barely. I was slowly but surely erasing myself. There were months when my electric bill was less than twenty dollars. Don't need any lights to lie on the couch. I was in hibernation.

A good day was when I managed to get out of bed before noon and brush my teeth and hair. Not once did it occur to me that I was exhibiting the textbook symptoms of depression. Profoundly painful dejection? Check. Cessation of interest in the outside world? Check. Inhibition of all activity? Check. I began to entertain thoughts of ending my life, and it still didn't register that anything could be clinically wrong with me. I just thought I was worthless. Useless. Past my expiration date. I imagined checking out early and nobody finding my body until the landlord came around to collect the rent. In my mind, suicidal ideation was a perfectly reasonable response to my escalating issues: my isolation, my inertia, my weight gain.

Obviously, my weight gain was noticeable when I was at the

rink. To the best of my knowledge, nobody paused to consider that there might be something behind my packing on the pounds beyond a lack of willpower. The cause-effect relationship seemed clear: *She overate and got fat.* It's incredible that nobody considered the effect-cause angle: *What's going on that led her to put on all that weight?*

Toward the end of spring, Carly flew to Detroit for a long weekend. She presented it as a girls' weekend, but it really was an intervention. I hadn't kept in great touch with her, which was shocking to anyone who knew us. We had been drifting apart since she retired from skating. By the middle of 2017 my id wanted nothing to do with her superego. I was mad at her for her role in keeping family secrets from me, and for what I also perceived as her dereliction of duty in choosing to take care of herself over helping me manage Mom's decline. I couldn't see then that she was establishing healthy boundaries while trying to navigate the real world, college, and a social life.

I just felt abandoned.

Her visit was painful for both of us. It was clear to Carly that I was seriously unwell. She had heard from coaches that I wasn't coming to the rink, but to see the evidence of my physical decline up close was jarring. The situation was precarious. She waited until the last day of her visit to have a heart-to-heart talk. Her basic message, as I remember it, was, *Gracie, can you please get your shit together because Mom and Dad are flying off the rails?* She pleaded with me to have a relationship with Mom and lose weight "just to make it easier."

Looking back, I see that Carly was in an impossible spot, caught between her fucked-up parents and her flailing sister. She was managing Mom on her own for the first time and reeling from Dad's shocking job loss while juggling the demands of college. When she came to Detroit and barely recognized me, the person she knows best in this world, she was completely shaken. It says a lot about where we were as a family that she determined I was the easiest one to "fix," though she had no clue how to go about it. It would have been a tall task for the most qualified therapist. It was asking way too much of Carly, who couldn't carry the weight of our family's struggles anymore. Her superglue could no longer hold together our fraying lives.

If she was harsh with me, it was out of desperation. She needed my cooperation to save our family from falling totally apart. But I wasn't open to anything she had to say. We had a massive fight. We were twenty-one years old and managing situations way beyond our expertise. Both of us were on the verge of tears when she summoned an Uber driver for the ride to the airport. Carly had shot her best shot and it had been an airball. We were more estranged than ever. Several weeks passed before we spoke again.

Meanwhile, my condition continued to deteriorate. I had lost my appetite for skating months ago and now I was losing my zest for life. Anger and sadness overwhelmed me. My whole identity was tied up in skating. If I wasn't a skater, why should I continue to exist? For the first time, I could understand why people feel like death is the preferable option.

Whenever I found myself pondering in a vague sort of way a permanent exit strategy, I thought of Carly and reeled back the impulse. The fact that we weren't on good terms made it even more imperative that I stick around for her. No matter how great my pain, I would not leave Carly and risk her feeling consumed by guilt wondering what she could have said or done differently during her visit to Detroit to help me. Our next communication came in the summer when I texted her after my demise was given a name. Well, two, actually: depression and trauma.

14

NUCLEAR MELTDOWN

I slouched on the ice, a sorry sight in my oversized black hoodie and black leggings. My uncombed hair resembled a rat's nest, and my face was mostly makeup free. I couldn't be bothered even to apply a swipe of my signature lipstick, CoverGirl Lip Perfection Hot 305, and just looking at my eyeliner pen exhausted me. For me, gliding onto the ice without lipstick was like a cop reporting for duty without a bulletproof vest. Makeup was part of the armor that steeled me for competition.

It was six months from my arranged date with destiny at the Olympics in Pyeongchang, South Korea, and I was, to put it mildly, a mess. For more than a year, it had been easier to deny my despair than dig down to its origins. But as summer waned, my deterioration was so pronounced, I couldn't pretend any longer.

I saw my depression and anxiety and weight gain as the universe's way of telling me to move along. I was being extended a cosmic vaudeville hook. It was time for me to leave the stage.

Quiet exits had never really been my scene, though. Predictably, I became more sullen, more self-indulgent.

The fact that I was extended an invitation to Champs Camp, an elite pre-season boot camp, after my lackluster performances during the 2016–17 season was inexplicable. More puzzling was that I bothered to show up. My mindset was that Outofshape-worthlessloser would make an appearance, everybody would see how far gone I was, I'd get kicked off the national team, and that would be the last anybody heard of or from me. To be clear, I didn't have a suicide plan drawn up in my head. But that doesn't mean I wasn't at the point where I couldn't see playing out my sad life indefinitely—maybe just until my money ran out, which wouldn't have taken much longer.

The camp was held that year in Colorado Springs, where U.S. Figure Skating is headquartered. The mile-high altitude was the least of my worries. I hadn't landed a clean triple in over six months, had gained over fifty pounds, and had largely sworn off basic grooming standards.

What could possibly go wrong?

I challenge you to find anybody who would truthfully say that they like Champs Camp. It's a device employed by U.S. Figure Skating to track our progress heading into a new season. We perform our programs, and officials can see how committed (or not) we were to training during our so-called offseason. I couch it that way because are we really getting time "off" when our months between the end of one season and the start of the next are spent crisscrossing the globe doing ice shows? It is a recipe for burnout, but no matter. We are expected to show up at Champs Camp recharged and raring to go. I never looked forward to attending, but like the good little overachiever I prided myself on being, I always showed up ready and performed respectably.

For that reason alone, my August 2017 appearance raised

enough red flags to line a downhill ski run. The Gracie Gold who had once bantered with Jay Leno and baked with Taylor Swift was long gone. In her place was a pucker-faced depressive. I was north of 170 pounds, and nobody, but *nobody,* was comparing me to Grace Kelly.

And yet, instead of wondering what might be going on in my life to trigger such a physical transformation, the men running U.S. Figure Skating gave off a distinct vibe that I was flipping the bird to the sport in some willful, and increasingly tiresome, act of rebellion. It was not unlike how the men in Hollywood treated the pop star Britney Spears and the socialite Paris Hilton, two high-profile women I grew up admiring whose private struggles were milked for the public's entertainment. They drew derision for being spoiled rich girls instead of sympathy for their vulner-abilities. When I was twelve or thirteen, I remember seeing a tabloid story that described how the singer Jessica Simpson, a contemporary of Hilton and Spears, was "packing on the pounds" when she was a size six. It's the sports and entertainment world's answer to the madonna/whore complex. You're either spoiled or a centerfold.

There seemed to be a fundamental lack of understanding that I wasn't sad because I hadn't won a stupid World Championships medal. I was sad because the sport and the system seemed rigged against its athletes. It pissed me off that people couldn't see that. I resented that the people who should care about my well-being didn't seem to be taking my deterioration seriously, which became a problem when they actually did reach out to help me. I was suspicious of their motives. If it's possible to be the face of a sport and be invisible, that's how I felt.

Everybody could see that I was unwell, but all that mattered was what wasn't right with my skating. I felt unsupported. Discarded like a broken skate lace. My value to U.S. Figure Skating could be summarized as: *When you're hot you're hot, and when you're not, you're nothing.* I'm aware that people in the organization would vehemently dispute my point of view. But if I'm exaggerating, why was I allowed to deteriorate for so long?

At the start of the camp I intended to go through the motions and offer my trained responses. You know, self-protection through sarcasm.

How am I doing, you ask? Oh, you know, living the dream.

I took to the ice looking like the Grim Reaper. I could feel the censorious stares of the skating officials bore through me. I didn't attempt a single triple, fell on a double Axel, and popped some of my other doubles. After my spins sputtered and my watered-down jumps landed with a thud, I faced my executioners on the panel. A few sat at the judges' table crying because my unraveling was so upsetting to them.

I'll never, ever forget the scathing critique delivered by one judge: "It seems like you've lost all respect for yourself."

Really? I'm at rock bottom, literally on the verge of not existing, and that's your hot take?

One of the officials, whose wife had gone through inpatient treatment, recognized a lot of her in my behavior. He was apparently the first to broach the idea of rehab. It didn't register with me because my head exploded when someone said, "Gracie, when the student is ready, the teacher will appear." *What. The. Fuck. What does that even mean, and how is it even remotely applicable to my current state of being?* It was such a complete misreading of the situation. I registered it as the most toxic example of tough love that I've experienced.

That comment was the final indignity. I was in the throes of a mental health crisis, and they were acting like I was throwing myself a pity party. I snapped. Acquiescent Gracie gave way to Angry Gracie. I could no longer even pretend to be a good foot soldier (though federation officials would probably argue that I never really was). What happened next could best be described as the mother of all meltdowns. I fired a fusillade of f-bombs at the panel. I was sobbing. A river of snot was running down my face. I. Did. Not. Care. At one point I distinctly remember screaming, "Can't anybody see the cry for help that is my existence right now?"

I probably could have phrased my words more delicately. I felt at the time that anger was my only power source, so I might as well plug into it. My skating had been going sideways for so long. It was disheartening to finally sacrifice myself at the altar of vulnerability and have U.S. Figure Skating officials act like I was just an attention-seeking drama queen.

This I recall with absolute clarity: I was informed that if I lost thirty pounds in the next two months my fall Grand Prix assignments, which were being rolled back, would be restored. Left unsaid was how I was expected to lose thirty pounds in two months in a healthy manner.

I was excused from performing my short program because everybody had seen enough. That was fine by me. I had nothing to show the skating officials, and I didn't see the point of going back out there and further embarrassing myself. What did they want me to do? Say, *Please, sirs, may I do another program?* That was never going to happen.

I was beyond caring about this high-performance camp, beyond caring about my health. Beyond caring about anything. With no more programs to muddle through, I escaped to my dorm room. Where else was I going to go? The Garden of the Gods is a serene spot to sit with an existential crisis. Hiking trails abound in Colorado Springs, but getting to either of those would have required energy, exertion. Ambition. So they were out of the question. With nothing to do and nowhere to go and all day to get there, I made my way to the training center's kitchen. It's a beautiful, expansive space where I knew I'd find Susie, a sports dietitian and high-performance director.

Even though she has lived in the United States for many years, Susie has managed to keep her native Australian accent, and I found her stretched-out vowels as comforting as a bulky sweatshirt. She is an empathetic person who is excellent at her job. She recognized the connection between diet and brain health, diet and growth spurts, diet and injuries. I entered the kitchen to find Susie bustling around.

She asked me if I was interested in baking something. Sure, I said. I mean, why not? We got to work making trail mix cookies with sunflower seeds, something healthy but also palatable to the taste buds. Jen, a doctor who worked for U.S. Figure Skating, was keeping Susie company in the kitchen when I arrived. I liked Jen enormously. She was one of the few people who would ask me about my life outside of skating. Sure enough, as I was standing there, mostly watching Susie do her thing, Jen casually asked about my family. How was everybody doing?

"Oh, we're super awesome," I answered, which was very me. Easy, breezy, revealing nothing.

My way of deflecting discomfort is through dark humor, and perhaps it's an indication of how miserable I was in my own skin that I didn't stop there. I kept talking, my sentences spinning one way, then switching direction and going around and around like a conversational sit-spin.

"I'm actually not talking to anybody in my family. I'm not speaking to my mom at all. She's drinking pretty heavily and I don't know why, but it seems bad, and my dad stole drugs from the hospital where he was working and then he lost his job and so now I'm estranged from everybody and on my own and Carly isn't speaking to me because in some ways she feels that even though none of this

was my fault, I didn't do anything to help keep our family together. But on the bright side, I haven't killed myself yet, so things are going really well."

I exhaled. My breath came out as a laugh meant to take the edge off my words. My mom giggles when confronted with trauma and, unfortunately, it's one of her habits that I inherited. Jen didn't see what was so funny. As I spoke, the picture developed like a Polaroid in Jen's mind.

I could see the dawning of comprehension on her face: *That's why Gracie doesn't have her shit together. Her whole world has imploded. That's what's causing her to behave like she doesn't fucking care. That's why she's so unprepared and out of shape.*

I opened my mouth to apologize for burdening her with my problems. But then Jen began talking in a no-nonsense tone that stopped me short: "Gracie, what you're describing is trauma. This is not self-indulgence. This is a real mental health crisis."

With her words, Jen shattered the glass of the snow globe that I had been trapped in. The relief I felt was palpable. I had been seen. Jen had heard me. What a gift it was to present myself, warts and all, to someone and not have them run away or ignore me or scold me or make me feel like my problems were all in my head.

My suicidal ideation had been rooted in a vague notion that I could always check out early if I decided life had gotten bad enough and I couldn't handle it anymore. I never had a concrete plan. I looked at death like an unhappily married couple looks at divorce: It was always there, lurking, as an option if the going got too tough and the pain became unbearable. I didn't really want to die. I just couldn't continue to live the way that I was, which probably helps explain my moment of candor in the kitchen. From somewhere deep inside me, a small voice urged me to tell someone what was going on before it was too late.

Receiving validation that my problems were not in my head

but were, in fact, reasonable responses to excessive stress helped me to reframe how I looked at my situation. I didn't need to feel ashamed and embarrassed to be taking up space in the world. I was not fundamentally fucked up. My circumstances were fucked up. And my external situation would be a lot easier to change than who I was at my core. The warmth I felt was a glimmer of light penetrating the darkness.

Jen reached out to Brandon, the strength and conditioning coach for the USOPC. I adored Brandon. Like Jen, he also had made the effort over the years to actively invest in me, the person. Whenever I was in Colorado Springs for something skating-related, he'd say to me, "We're going hiking." I'm not really a trails-and-camping kind of chick, and by this time my agoraphobia was in full flower. But I loved my walks with Brandon because we'd exercise our mouths as much as our legs. We'd talk about everything but skating. He'd been working with me on a fitness plan, but after Jen told him what was going on with me, he shifted gears and researched recovery centers. I've heard Mitch say that treatment was his idea, but my recollection is that Brandon did most of the legwork in finding me a facility. That said, I don't doubt that I have Mitch to thank for U.S. Figure Skating and the USOPC footing the $50,000 bill, though at the time I was so discombobulated that it didn't occur to me to ask who was picking up the tab.

I owe so much to Jen and Susie and Brandon. I look at them as real-life guardian angels. I shudder to think what would've become of me if they hadn't intervened. Thank goodness they brought a holistic approach to their work, one that didn't discard the person in service to the performance.

When presented with the offer of inpatient rehab, I wish I could say that I immediately recognized the lifeline being extended to me. I did not. Not automatically. We were near the end of an Olympic cycle, which gave me pause. With the 2018 Winter Games six months off, was it really wise to completely disrupt my schedule to check into a recovery center for six weeks? It was ludicrous for me to think the Olympics were still on the table. But the lies we tell ourselves to live die hard.

I replayed my disastrous free skate in my mind. That gave me the clarity I needed. I wasn't competitive anyway, so why not give this rehab thing a try? If I didn't like it or it wasn't working out, I could always check out. There was a quote that I wrote down in my journal: "If you don't heal the cut, you'll bleed on people who didn't hurt you." I thought of the people I had metaphorically bled on: Carly, Mom, Frank.

Between receiving the offer and registering my response, maybe thirty seconds or a minute went by. A flash, really, but time enough for the universe to deliver a realization that permeated my defenses and defied my stubborn disposition: *If my downfall is upsetting to people, they must care about me on some level, and if they care about me on some level, I must not be worthless, and if I'm not worthless, then maybe, just maybe, whatever's broken and buried deep inside me can be fixed.*

In a burst of courage, I replied, "Sure. Sign me up." (I've since learned that Mitch Moyer has described that moment as one of the happiest days of his life.)

On some level I understood that insanity is doing the same thing over and over and expecting a different result. I knew I needed to change, and I recognized that if my life got any worse, I was going to wind up dead. And I realized, somewhat to my astonishment, that I wanted to live. I leaned in to the joke told by the comic Sarah Silverman: Suicide is best put off until tomorrow.

Looking back, I can see that showing up at Champs Camp was my cry for help. Thank God there were people with big hearts who heard me, who didn't roll their eyes and say, "You have the whole package. What do you have to be depressed about?"

When Jen and Susie and Brandon assured me that I actually was sick and that there were resources to help me, I felt relief—but also vindication. In accepting their help, I was blowing a raspberry at all the skating officials, coaches, judges, and others who had disparaged my work ethic and questioned my self-respect. Who had called me a mess. A disaster. A lazy ass. Who had lectured me to get my shit together. To grow up. To snap out of it. I trust they got the message: *I'm getting admitted to an inpatient facility because I'm considering checking out of this world early. Do you guys all feel like shit now for being so heartless and careless about the athletes you pretend to care about?*

With the assistance of my management team, I issued a statement saying that I was stepping away from skating to seek professional help. Not for nothing, my announcement came less than a week after one of my Russian rivals, nineteen-year-old Yulia Lipnitskaya, retired after spending three months in treatment for anorexia. My statement began:

> My passion for skating and training remains strong. However, after recent struggles on and off the ice, I realize I need to seek some professional help and will be taking some time off while preparing for my Grand Prix assignments. This time will help me become a stronger person, which I believe will be reflected in my skating performances as well.

I wanted to spell out the specifics of my leave-taking. But there were risk-averse sponsors to appease. And competition judges whose minds needed to be kept open in case I was able to start my season, as scheduled, in Japan in October, and honor my Grand Prix assignments in China and France the following month.

I never believed those competitions were going to happen for me, but I was fine playing along.

It was only after it became obvious to everyone else that I was going to be in no shape to skate anytime soon that a second, more transparent release was drafted, one that squashed all the rumors that had rushed in to fill the information void after I entered treatment—including my favorite, *Gracie's pregnant!* It stated that I was pulling out of all my competitions for the rest of the year because I was being treated for depression, anxiety, and an eating disorder.

It wasn't the time to worry about my marketability. It was time for me to lay down my defenses before it was too late. The second statement buried the news: that by forgoing the competitions, I was essentially forfeiting any shot at a 2018 Olympic team berth, since I wouldn't be able to fulfill all the competitive requirements for consideration.

"It saddens me deeply to sit out this Grand Prix Series," I said in the statement, "but I know it is for the best."

And then I dropped off the face of the earth.

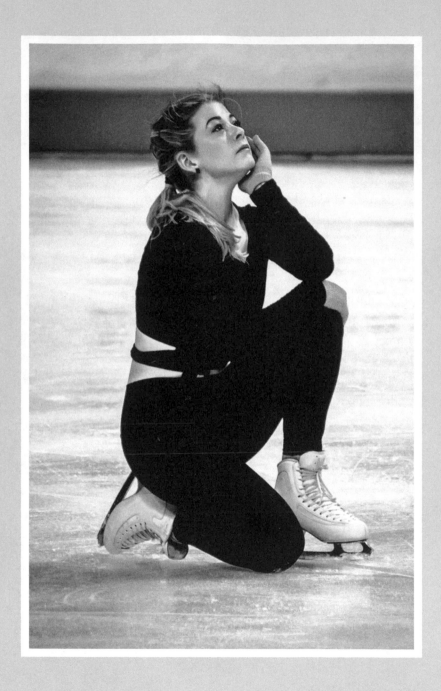

ME

PART FOUR

Maybe the journey isn't so much about becoming
anything. Maybe it's about unbecoming
everything that isn't really you, so you can be
who you were meant to be in the first place.

—PAULO COELHO

15

MOTHS ALWAYS FIND THE LIGHT

Not to say that I was clueless about what I was signing up for when I agreed to inpatient treatment at The Meadows, but in my journal I described it as a "forty-five-day cleanse." Like my days were going to be filled with colonics and protein shakes.

My wake-up call came at check-in, when I was asked to extend an arm for a blood draw and to submit to a tuberculosis shot because illicit drug users are at a greater risk of TB. Oh, and to provide a urine sample for a pregnancy test. The technicians were unmoved by my argument that I had been exclusively dating a woman for much of the past year.

I was asked to relinquish my phone, my books, and all of my electronics, including my hair dryer, because anything with a long cord could be used, in theory, to hang myself. And yet the here-and-now struck me as less precarious than the future. I distinctly remember wondering what would happen when I got my phone back and turned it on. Would it blow up with calls and messages? What if no one had tried to contact me? How would I survive if my phone stirred to life as quietly as an electric car?

On the intake application, I listed disordered eating as my pre-senting issue. It never occurred to me to include depression. For my first twenty-two years, I believed that if you were depressed, the cure was to tough it out. Go to the gym. Sign up for an extra cycling class. Schedule an extra session on the ice. Exercise to exorcise your demons.

I assumed you entered treatment only for substance- or food-related addictions. Sadness, to me, was part of the human condition—the flip side of happiness. And if "sadness" was a word that often fit me like a crop top, falling well short of cover-ing my depression, well, I figured, that's what happens when you have big feelings. While our culture had finally started to accept a broader range of body types, I hadn't seen many accommoda-tions being made for plus-size emotions.

I accepted as gospel the saying "Tough times don't last, but tough people do." I considered any mental health struggle to be a sign of weakness. It probably was a blessing that I thought that I was signing up for a forty-five-day cleanse. If I had known that I'd be required to sit with my vulnerability at The Meadows, I doubt I would have gone through the front door.

I checked in on the last day of August, and it was hotter than hell in Wickenburg, Arizona, the tumbleweed town where the center is located. Dry heat, my ass. I stepped outside and my plas-tic Barbie-doll face melted. That first day, I would have told you that I'd stay for one week. Two weeks tops.

I had this vague idea that I'd check in, meet with a therapist to say that I had, then leave after a week or two, in time to skate in one or two of my assigned competitions to prepare for the Olym-pics. My denial ran deep. Fortunately, I also had a germ of a belief that whatever this experience held, it had to be an improvement over my current situation, which was pretty grim. I had lost that voice in my head that always pushed me to keep moving, to persist. I went to The Meadows to recover it.

As soon as I walked through the door, I realized: *There are a lot of rules here.* No caffeine was one of them, and it was a literal headache, given that I had pretty much been subsisting on vanilla soy lattes and was now in full withdrawal. No shoelaces were allowed, either, for the same reason that anything with a long cord was strictly forbidden. It was clear that patients were not to be trusted.

From 7 a.m. breakfast to 10 p.m. lights-out, our days were highly structured. We had time set aside for therapy sessions, for exercise, for meals. My first impression was that I was in the wrong place. I found myself among people who had parole officers or heroin addictions. What could I possibly have in common with "Meth Girl," who blinked with only one eye? I felt like a little angel next to some of the kids.

My second impression was that first impressions can be misleading.

After the first few days of group therapy sessions, I could feel a shift in my attitude. It was as if I had found a safe shelter from the swirling shitstorm that was the outside world. I recognized I was exactly where I needed to be. The other kids were just like me. I was no better or worse than anyone else.

An aha moment came when I connected the dots between my erratic eating and my yo-yoing emotions. I knew my relationship with food was completely fucked up, and that didn't change right away at The Meadows. I mostly ate Grape-Nuts cereal and peanut-butter-and-honey sandwiches, which I washed down with water infused with Crystal Light powder or iced tea sweetened with Splenda. I have a weakness for carrot cake, so I felt strong when I was able to refrain from grabbing a piece when it was on the menu, in which case I noted it in my journal with a little "Yay, me." If I caved, it was a tragedy. "RIP diet," I'd write, and chastise myself for not choosing tea with honey if I was craving something sweet. I'd failed to exert discipline over my eating yet again, and that's why I was depressed—or so I thought. But during my sessions, I gradually came to understand that it could be the other way around: that maybe my depression came first and fed my eating issues. It was one of many clarifying moments I experienced during my stay.

What a relief it was to learn that it's okay if you don't wake up every day feeling hopeful or excited about the future. That's normal. You don't have to look for nonexistent sunshine and rainbows or pretend to be fine when you're not. Sometimes it's enough to be curious about what lies ahead. I was drawn to rehab by the promise of something different on the horizon.

I was diagnosed with severe depression, anxiety, and moderate obsessive-compulsive disorder. I was one personality disorder diagnosis short of a bingo on my bonkers card. It was a lot to process. The OCD should not have come as any surprise to someone who avoids cracks in the sidewalk and whose intrusive thoughts spawned an entire persona, Outofshapeworthlessloser.

But in truth, I was a little taken aback. I had always considered my love of order a personality trait, not a coping mechanism. I made sure all my pink blouses and shirts hung in a row because I was a neatnik, not to soothe myself after an upsetting turn of events.

I was prescribed Prozac, starting with 10 milligrams a day and topping out at 50 milligrams. I took it faithfully during my time in treatment but found that it made my insomnia a hundred times worse, which I hadn't thought possible. I ended up quitting it cold turkey, which you're not supposed to do, and I understood why after I got this weird tremor in my right hand, a spasm in my jaw, and profuse sweats. Once I was in a better headspace, I decided to slowly taper off it, because the tremor and spasm were working against the pill's intended effects—they freaked me out.

My forty-five days in treatment felt like a much-needed time-out from my life. I had no pressure. No expectations. No need to perform for anybody. Gone was any expectation of squeezing the maximum productivity out of every waking hour, an intention that I was accustomed to carrying into every day. Slowly, I took back the life that skating had stolen from me as a child.

I learned the value of stillness. Of silliness. I learned to let go of the illusion that my life could have, or should have, been any different. After so many years spent in skating's cookie-cutter culture, I reveled in being part of this community of imperfect people. We learned a saying in treatment that has become my mantra: *If you replace the "i" with "we," illness becomes wellness.*

As the days went on, I could feel Gracie Gold receding into the shadows. Outofshapeworthlessloser grew fainter, too, and someone new began to assert herself. It was thrilling. I can't remember what part of my therapy triggered it, but I can distinctly recall being struck by this thought: *Oh, there's some real substance here.*

For someone invested in building walls to hide her real self, the group therapy sessions were a revelation. It was wonderful to be surrounded by people who understood what I was going through, possibly better than I did. Nobody in the group circle accused me of laziness or self-sabotage. From listening to everyone else's stories, I recognized that my behaviors were not about self-destruction. They were about maintaining an illusion of control. It was liberating to hear patients articulate the hurt I was feeling but had never been able to express. And it was refreshing to hear the therapists talk about pain not as something to be avoided at all costs but as a path to profound change. I knew to embrace the physical pain in skating from fatigue or falls, but until treatment I hadn't made the connection that emotional pain can also be a harbinger of growth.

There was a social aspect to treatment that gave me a taste of the college experience I had passed up for skating. I woke up my roommate some mornings by jumping on her bed. I organized "spa" sessions where I'd give the other girls facials. I cleaned up a *lot* of eyebrows. I bonded with kids over loads of laundry or tarot card readings, and I spent mealtimes talking with my new friends about everything on our minds. I hadn't enjoyed that kind of easy, breezy companionship since my days hanging out in the school cafeteria with the theater geeks in Springfield, Illinois.

After years of striving to separate myself from everybody else—of having "extraordinary" be the baseline of my existence—to be seen and treated as nothing special was wonderful. Nobody knew me as an Olympic figure skater. (No one except for Jen from the USOPC, who visited multiple times, which I appreciated.) When I was asked what I did, I said I liked to skate and left it at that. Nobody had access to the internet to fill in the details. The jig was up during family week, when one of my friends went off campus with her parents and entered my name into a search engine on her mother's phone. Upon her return, she found me and said, "Gracie, you really undersold this skating thing of yours."

To be liked for who I was, as is, was huge. I couldn't remember the last time I had been accepted for being a good person as opposed to a great athlete. When I was eight, maybe? It was mind-blowing to realize that Outofshapeworthlessloser, who believed I was a fraud and a garbage human, was not speaking for the majority. In fact, I was shocked to find out that she was a party of one. In a notebook that people signed on my "graduation day," I was described as "funny and brilliant" and "a huge ray of sunshine" and "an amazing, kind, loving person." Multiple people commented on how I was "always smiling and laughing." Maybe the best compliment I received was from the young woman who said I was one of the "realest and baddest bitches" she'd ever met.

I was surrounded by people who did not hide their failures because of any shame of falling short of expectations. All of us were in recovery because we were not thriving. There was no sense pretending otherwise. The people I met at The Meadows had no preconceived ideas about me that got in the way of us genuinely connecting. I could gain a friend by offering to throw their laundry in with mine, or by giving them a facial, or by just sitting with them while they had a good cry. Being a decent, empathetic, real human being was enough.

Slowly, a person emerged in treatment who might have been me if skating hadn't turned me into someone else. A "bad bitch" who loved whaling on a punching bag in the gym in the morning and practicing tai chi at night. It felt good to hit that bag with all my might. It made me feel *alive*. Not on autopilot like when I did my carefully counted spins, precise jumps, and set step sequences.

I ventured far out of my comfort zone to play in sand volleyball matches. Or as we described it, "adult recess." There was more shit talk than rallies. It was amazing. One time I accidentally got smacked hard in the face with the ball, leaving an angry red welt, which I proudly referred to as my battle scar. It was exhilarating because no one was concerned that my nose or teeth might have gotten messed up and how that would impact my skating. All that mattered was we won the point after the ball ricocheted off my face and into the reach of my friend, who spiked a winner. *Take that, you plastic-faced phony!*

We spent a lot of time outdoors at The Meadows. I loved it. I'd spent so much of my life under the artificial lights of a rink, I had forgotten how much I liked being in the sunshine. I ventured out to the pool. It was the first time I had been in a swimsuit in public in almost a year. I was self-conscious about my huge chest, and overall size, but I felt surprisingly okay because I didn't feel like I was being judged by anybody (you know, besides myself).

At the end of my second week, I participated in a session that was fucking awesome. I was able to tell my story, to give voice to every resentment I had against my parents. I was surprised by the intensity of my anger. I'd been stuffing it down for years because I'd believed that ugly outbursts are for children and conflict is stressful and dramatic and to be avoided at all costs. The rage shot out of me like a geyser.

How I was never allowed to do anything fun.

How I never got even five minutes to myself to reset or decompress when I was upset.

How my entire childhood was highly structured and over-scheduled.

How, if Carly and I had not been Mom's shields against Dad, and our success had not served as our parents' barometer of their success, I might have been able to view my skating achievements as wonderful instead of as necessary to keep the family going.

How we lacked any semblance of stability during my teenage years, moving from one city to another, ostensibly for my skating, but with the fringe benefit of my mother gaining physical separation from my dad.

How Dad always told us of his boundless love for his family, but then went out and had relationships with other women. What did those other women have that his wife and daughters couldn't provide?

Around this time, I wrote letters to both my parents as part of a therapeutic exercise. I would read them aloud in group, but my parents wouldn't see them, so I held nothing back. I expressed disappointment in my dad. "Dear Dad," I wrote, in part,

Your behavior has been inexcusable and you're finally seeing the repercussions of it. I'm glad. I want that to stare you in the face. I'm frustrated because I'm conflicted. You weren't directly a "bad dad," but you were absent a lot and sometimes so angry I was beyond scared. But knowing what I know about your addictions and your behavior, it's hard for me to look at you the same as I used to.

I directed most of my rage at my mom. "Dear Mother," I began, and then crossed out "Mother" and wrote "Denise" in its place, the formality signaling that my kid gloves were well and truly off. I told her that I knew that 99 percent of the time she had meant well but her actions, nonetheless, had caused Carly and me so much pain and anxiety and distress. And how we couldn't talk to her about it because she invariably started sobbing and apologizing.

Growing up was hard. The intense pressure and expectations from you, myself, and everyone else has almost killed me. There was never a moment where I could just be myself and not Gracie Gold.

My skating controlled your life and therefore our lives. The chaos and crazy that we lived in within our home was exhausting. Not to mention all the other shit life threw at us. I know life has been hard for you—it's thrown you too many bad hands to count. But that's why we need help now. Before we both implode for good.

It's never too late to be the best version of yourself. To be the person you've always wanted to become.

My mom and I call to mind the irresistible-force paradox. I'm the irresistible force and she's the immovable mass, which means our relationship is characterized by conflicts for which there are no logical resolutions. I know Mom felt guilty that I'd ended up in recovery. She sent me care packages stuffed with cosmetics and clothing. I recognized those gifts for what they were: her peace offering to express how sorry she was about everything. No need to apologize. I know she was coming from a place of generosity, trying to give me and Carly all the support and resources that she'd missed out on as a child. She truly did the best she could. As my default parent, Mom bore the brunt of all my big feelings. I could unload my rage at her feet because I knew she wasn't going anywhere. That I let my dad off the hook, relatively speaking, didn't mean that I wasn't infuriated by his behavior. It's just that I had come to expect less from him in general.

I was ready to build an identity outside of my disordered eating, which had been a part of my life longer than most of my inner circle. I knew it wouldn't be easy. My food issues, however destructive, had served a purpose. As long as my energies were focused on my diet, I didn't have to confront my parents or unpack my emotional baggage. Shortly after I wrote those letters, I decided it was time to stop avoiding the truth.

Mom and Dad traveled to Arizona from their respective homes to participate in family week. By then, I had untangled some of my crossed wires. I recognized that saying "I feel fat" or "I'm out of shape" was easier than giving voice to what was really gnawing at me, like "I'm afraid I can't live up to the expectations people have for me" or "I'm anxious about my parents' relationship."

I looked forward to sharing these insights with my mom and dad. I hoped to establish an open line of communication with them. I didn't expect either to be 100 percent honest with me, but I figured they would be brutally honest with me about each other. Neither disappointed me in that regard. I'd have breakfast with my father and he'd go off on my mother. I'd have lunch with my mother and she'd unload on my father. Family week is when I found out Dad had been married before. And that he had been to treatment for his addictions before Carly and I were born. We knew from comments made by Mom over the years that he had struggled with alcohol, but we had had no idea to what extent—or that prescription pills were also a problem for him. The pieces of the puzzle started to click into place.

As a small child, I was frightened by my dad's temper. Every day I worried about doing or saying something to trigger his next blowup. During the last year and a half of my time in Southern California, I'd entertained the same worries about my mom. Her demons surfaced when she drank too much and scared me shit-less. I've heard mental disorders described as a complex equation that is 60 percent genetics and 40 percent environment, with the environment typically triggering the genetic component.

I had carried around a sizable amount of guilt over my parents' unhappy marriage. I blamed my skating for pulling them apart. The story I told myself was that if our family had remained phys-ically intact, we all would have been so much better off. Life would have been a fucking Norman Rockwell painting. In family week an alternative picture emerged. My mother and father had a fucked-up relationship with or without my skating. My dad's addictions probably doomed my parents' marriage before they officially became husband and wife.

They are much better together when they are mostly apart, and in that respect, their legal union, such as it is, has survived to this day because they've led separate lives for most of the last two decades.

I began to better understand how I had ended up where I did. Because my parents hid their addictions from me and Carly, we essentially inherited a GPS with the destination already entered, only it was somewhere we didn't want to go, and we had no idea why it was taking us there.

Encouraged by the insights I gained in therapy, I would later lose myself in research, reading studies that provided further clarity (and also put me off ever wanting to have children of my own). One hit especially close to home. It showed that having too little money can be detrimental to happiness. But owing to the toxic effects of aspiration and acquisition, so can scaling the income ladder beyond the point of financial stability. I think parenting operates similarly. Too little of a parent's attention and the child will greatly suffer. But too much of a parent's attention can also adversely impact the child, who ends up feeling smothered, controlled, incompetent.

The parenting sweet spot—that space between being too involved and too hands-off—is so hard to find. It becomes nearly impossible when your child is a prodigy or, in my case, an Olympian, and your husband has addiction issues.

I spent years believing that there was something I could say or do, something I might accomplish in skating that would magically change my parents into the people I wanted them to be. In treatment, I let go of those hopes and undertook the excruciating work of shedding my expectations and accepting my mom and dad as they are. During family week I made a collage as part of our art therapy. I attempted to capture in images what I had expressed in words in those unsent letters. Using the art room's child-safe scissors, I cut out clippings from magazines and arranged them on construction paper, toiling away until my fingers were covered in the nontoxic, anti-self-harm glue and my inner child was satisfied that the finished piece conveyed the feelings she had kept bottled up.

At the center was me, "the family gift." I clipped the phrase "no boundaries" from a magazine to represent my mother, who took it upon herself to fix my problems and clear obstacles in my path without realizing how damaging that was to my sense of competence. For my father, I cut out a photo of Donald Trump and captioned it "monster."

All the culling of images, all the cutting and pasting and arranging everything just so on the oversized construction paper, helped me work through my complicated feelings and show my family as it was, not as we had projected it to be for years and years. I laid out on paper all of the things I had always felt but had never had the balls or the vocabulary to express. With that collage, I came out, if you will, as a person separate from the skater who was the family jewel. It was a poster proclaiming my independence. And I wasn't done.

Before I left The Meadows, I took a sheet of lined notebook paper and handwrote a press release that I would have liked to have seen U.S. Figure Skating send out before I dropped out of sight. I knew it wouldn't be seen by the public. The point was for me to take control of my narrative:

> It pains me deeply to sit out this Grand Prix Series, but I know that it is for the best. I am currently in treatment for depression, anxiety, suicidal ideation, and an eating disorder. I will not have adequate training time to prepare and compete at the level that I want to. I want to thank my federation, my fans, and my sponsors for their never-ending support. I also want to thank Marina and Oleg for taking me under their wing and inviting me into their skating family, and my family for their unconditional love. Thanks. —Gracie.

The mask hadn't totally dropped. I still felt the need to be a good girl and express gratitude that I didn't necessarily feel in the moment. But the mask was askew.

On my post-recovery to-do lists I addressed head-on the question *Where do I go from here?*

It was a scary proposition, leaving the cocoon of recovery. I knew that the growth I had experienced during the past forty-five days would mark the end of some relationships because there were people in my life who were more comfortable with the mentally ill version of me.

I was still in treatment when I broke up with Ellen, who hadn't wanted me to go to rehab in the first place. Was she worried that if I got better, we would have less in common? In therapy, I was forced to sit with the possibility that our demons had been what bonded us. Our angry outbursts—however "normal" to me—were scary, and our lack of boundaries precluded me from honoring my own. I had no idea who I was, but if I was going to find out, I needed to create distance from her.

I listed all the steps I hoped to take in the next few months:

Return to California.
Move in with Carly and her boyfriend.
Apply to colleges with an eye toward medical school.
Find the courage to be disliked.
Stay free and fearless in my authenticity and vulnerability.

A fresh start was in order. I didn't see how I could be my true self and return to a world that knew and revered Gracie Gold. Skating was off the table. I was so done with it. Knowing how much work I'd have to put in, for what would almost certainly be diminishing returns, I didn't see the point. The mere thought of returning to the rink was daunting, to say the least. But before I could move forward, I was required to continue my recovery as an outpatient while living with several others in a sober house in Scottsdale, Arizona.

We had household responsibilities, like vacuuming and dusting, which we determined by the spin of a chore wheel. If someone neglected their task, I'd step in and do it gladly. Cleaning became my new coping mechanism, a way of bringing physical order to my life. I attended group therapy sessions for five hours a day, Monday through Thursday, but beyond that, my waking hours seemed to stretch forever.

One night, my friend Cat (not her real name) and I decided to fill a few of those hours by going to a body piercing parlor. I got my septum pierced. It's not to be confused with an exterior nose piercing, which is child's stuff next to the badassery of allowing a needle to thread the piece of flesh toward the front of your nose, beyond the cartilage. Septum piercings are especially popular in the queer/alternative community. I realized I was opening myself up to judgment, but I didn't care. I personally thought I looked great with it.

After I was done, I watched as Cat got her nipples pierced. Cat's blood was everywhere. It looked like a goddamn crime scene. Not as in one of my poorly executed programs. Like *for real*. I don't consider myself squeamish in the least, but I had to look away.

Another night, I traded in my tight bun for a short bob haircut and decided to dye my hair brown to return my hair as close to its natural color as possible. What? You thought I was a natural blonde? Have you not seen my (exquisitely groomed) eyebrows?

I also acquired my first tattoo. I had never wanted the Olympic rings inked on my body. It was a popular rite of passage for Olympians in other sports, but it seemed frowned upon in skating. That I got any kind of tat was a shocking act of rebellion. From a young age, both my parents, but especially my dad, drilled into us that body ink was "bad" or "tasteless."

I credit a friend I made at The Meadows, let's call her Iris, for helping me see the light. She was a little older than me, but the shit she had seen and experienced made me wonder if she wasn't on her fifth or sixth life. She was in recovery for depression exacerbated by post-traumatic stress disorder. During a stint in the military, she had been sexually assaulted. Later, as an emergency medical technician, she had worked music festivals, which brought her into contact with revelers who overdosed on drugs. Some she couldn't revive.

We would meet in the courtyard, which we designated the "smoke pit"—it was near the women's dormitory and out of range of eavesdropping medical technicians—and puff on cigarettes. It was one of the few vices we were allowed. I thought it was a disgusting habit until I tried it. An entry in my journal from September 9, 2017, marked the occasion of my first cigarette. "I like them low-key," I wrote. Translation: *These are a hella good appetite suppressant.* By the time I got out of treatment, I was a full-fledged Marlboro Girl (and also a Newport Ninja), though I'd later switch to (and stay with) Juul vape pens, for which I'm sorry–not sorry. I feel like we all should be allowed one vice, and vaping is mine.

Iris and I would join a few others on a bench, or sometimes on the swings of an adult playset, and engage in spirited, and oftentimes profane, girl talk.

One day, I noticed that Iris had a sleeve of tattoos on her arm. They were beautiful. She pointed to a skull that she planned to have a skilled artist metamorphose into a moth.

"Why a moth?" I asked.

Iris replied, "They always find the light."

As she was talking, a large black moth fluttered around and landed on the middle of the table between us. It was a spooky moment. Later, it would occur to me that those bright porch lights that moths are inexorably drawn to are also the source of their destruction. Wow. What better metaphor for me and skating than a creature destroyed by the gravitational pull that it cannot resist?

During my unraveling, I had lost sight of the power of hope. And so after I left The Meadows, I got my own moth tattoo on my left side, on my rib cage. It was a bold choice for a first tattoo. Fun fact: It is very painful area to get tatted. I found out after the fact that it is one of the most sensitive spots on the body. So on-brand for me.

While these little rebellions were exciting, the halfway house also brought me back to reality. Cohabitating with people whose abuse of drugs or alcohol had landed them in recovery was a challenge. Some of my housemates were struggling with their re-entry into regular life. One or two relapsed while I was there. I felt like I was straddling two opposing shores, one solid and light-filled and inviting and the other porous and bleak and menacing. It became clear to me that for my own mental health, I needed to make my escape, find a job, ease my way back into regular society. The one thing I knew for certain is that Michigan was out of the picture. No way could I go back there. The mere thought of returning to the place of my unraveling made my stomach churn.

The Pyeongchang Olympics were all over the news. The Games I once hoped would serve as my coronation were taking place without me. I wasn't contemplating death anymore, but I didn't feel bracingly alive. Until I got a handle on my post-recovery life, I felt like it probably would be a good idea for multiple reasons if I stayed connected to the ice.

Who was I kidding? I was just another recovering addict in my halfway house who relapsed, only it wasn't obvious to anybody on the outside since my drug of choice, skating, is viewed as a healthy addiction. An admirable one, even.

Let's be real. Sport is the opiate of the elite athlete. Like the recovering alcoholic who insists that a little wine with dinner won't hurt, I told myself that I "wasn't like other addicts" and set out hoping that I could skate in moderation.

Could I be a figure skater without jeopardizing my mental and physical health? The road to answering that question has been difficult and strewn with some powerful—and painful—lessons.

16

SECOND ACT

My comeback was always going to be tricky. By sharing the story of my mental health struggles, I had put an ugly face on a beautiful sport. No longer could the public live in denial about the cost of excellence. In that respect, I had betrayed the covenant of skating: *Thou shalt not expose the pain behind the performance.*

Also, I wasn't sure exactly where I stood. Was I at the finish or the start? The lines became blurred when I needed a jump harness to afford me the hang time necessary to execute triples that once had come easily to me. Some people at the rink had no trouble making the distinction. In their eyes, I was done. Dusted. Kaput.

A teenage skater approached me between sessions one day and, in a tone more acidic than the coffee she held in her manicured hand, said, "Everyone thinks you're a clown."

ME: Oh. Okay. What do you want me to say to that?
HER: I mean, everyone in the locker room is shitting on you and thinks you skating again is such a joke.

ME: I don't really care what they think. I'm not going to argue
   with a bunch of teenagers.
HER: But aren't you so mad at them? Can you believe they are
   being such bitches about it? Don't worry. I'm not part of it.
ME: Well, it is what it is. I can't say I blame them.

Then I walked away. Bless her, but did she honestly believe I
was oblivious to the background noise? Did she think I was old
and deaf? I was well aware of what people were saying. Friends at
the rink had told me that mothers of other skaters were openly
disdainful of my presence. They huddled around a table in the
snack area on the other side of the plexiglass and whispered,
"Why is Gracie Gold still skating at her age?"

My sarcastic side was tempted to say, *However old and washed
up you think I am, I'm still better than your darling daughter.* But
I can't say I was bothered by any of the talk. I got it. It was very
bleak when I first started skating again. So many times in that
first year back I wanted to say, *Hey, can we all go easy on the fucking jokes, because I know better than anyone how this looks from
the outside?*

I kept largely silent because I had to agree with most of what
was being said. And though I wanted to, I couldn't articulate in
any artful way that the armchair criticism, coupled with the initial clumsiness, is probably why people don't bother trying to
come back to skating once they've been out of the sport for a
while—and certainly not when you're as far gone as I was.

What I was attempting was something far more difficult than
a quad. I was the first Olympian I knew of who was using inpatient treatment as a springboard to a competitive comeback. I
really, really wanted to prove that it was possible to do it.

But I'm not gonna lie. There's nothing more humbling than

being one of the worst girls at the rink. Especially when you used to be the best.

After months away from skating, you don't hop on the ice and effortlessly launch your body into the air. Most people couldn't comprehend why I'd open myself up to daily humiliations. Was my identity so tied up in skating that I couldn't move on and get a "real job"? To those who questioned my motivation, there was probably no satisfactory answer that I could give.

I was like Sisyphus pushing the boulder up the hill only to have it tumble back on me. That's a tragedy only if you see Sisyphus as a sucker circumscribed to spend eternity in a hopeless pursuit. Maybe I'm a masochist, but what the myth of Sisyphus meant to me was he was happy because he was doing his job. Like Sisyphus, I was happy to be doing my job, however grim it seemed.

More than anything, I wanted my skating to end on my terms. I didn't want my career to be like one of those acrimonious sport/athlete divorces that I've seen all too often, with skaters avoiding the rink and vowing never to let their offspring take up the sport because of how much they hated it by the end. I loved skating too much to spend the rest of my life resenting the hell out of it.

Also, I guess you could say that curiosity killed the quitter. I really wanted to find out: Could I be close to the skater that Gracie Gold was *and* a more honest version of myself?

My deep dive to find out began with an act of generosity by Vincent Restencourt, who emigrated from France and was coaching skaters at a rink outside Philadelphia, Pennsylvania, called IceWorks. Vincent was a fantastic jumping technician. During his competitive career in the nineties, he had become the first French skater to land a quad in competition. Wherever he went, the skaters he was working with quickly became noticeably more effective, efficient jumpers.

Vincent was introduced to me at the 2018 nationals by Mitch Moyer. His best skater at the time was a woman competing in juniors. That she was on her way up and I was on my way down didn't bother him at all. So enthusiastic was Vincent about my comeback, he offered to coach me for free. As they say, the price was right. At Mitch's suggestion, Vincent and Lisa, the IceWorks manager, reached out to me and arranged for me to coach several days of stand-alone private lessons. It was another offer that, given my financial circumstances, I couldn't refuse. I was on the next plane from Arizona to Pennsylvania, and I never looked back.

Everything I achieved in my second act I owe to Vincent, for bringing me to Philadelphia, and to a small group that includes Lisa and coaches Pavel (Pasha) Filchenkov and Alex Zahradnicek. They were the ones who cared enough to stop, pick up the pieces, and put me back together when I was a shattered human being whom most everyone else was stepping over or around without so much as a backward glance. Lisa, Pasha, and Alex believed in me when my faith in myself was shaky. Slowly but surely, they persuaded me that my talent wasn't like a pair of sunglasses left behind on an airplane and lost forever. My muscle memory still contained all that I needed to succeed.

These dear people have become more than my work colleagues. They're my chosen family, and I have unending gratitude for everything they've done for me. Pasha, in particular, I can't thank enough. There is no way I can ever pay him back for all that he has given me. His lack of judgment carried me through some dark days.

For an entire year, I let the coaches fasten me to a harness, held by Pasha, and talk me through what felt like literal leaps of faith. They worked with me two or three sessions a day with no promise that I'd ever return to competitive form. Their enthusiasm was contagious. As my jumps improved, I can remember Vincent posting videos of my best efforts to his social media accounts. He was creating a trail of evidence that, contrary to popular opinion, I had not fallen off the face of the earth.

Pasha, a retired ice dancer, forced me to confront the lies I'd been hiding behind for years to maintain a sense of control. If I was struggling with a jump, my default excuse was to blame my weight: I was "out of shape" or "not fit." Pasha's the only coach I've ever had who challenged that narrative. "Shut the fuck up!" he'd say, not unkindly. "That's not what's happening. Stop saying that. You're not fat. We know you can do this if you're lighter, but that's not the only reason you're struggling. You're just saying that because it's your escape so you don't have to talk about what's *really* bothering you."

Bingo. When my home life was unraveling in ways I couldn't fix, or I felt unprotected or vulnerable, I didn't know who it was safe to confide in, so I'd stiff-arm everybody and blame my weight. "I'm not in shape" was my version of "Whatever." It was a deflection, pure and simple, and Pasha, bless him, was the first to see through it. Thank God he did.

When I talk about wanting to be truly seen, that's what I mean. Other people in my life could say they cared and wanted to help me—and I don't doubt that they meant well—but if they took my behavior at face value, they were never going to get to the root of my problems. I'll be indebted to Pasha for meeting me where I was at and not backing down when I was trying my best to deflect.

Pasha believed in me, maybe to a fault. There would be times when I'd be on the verge of tears over something he wanted me to try. My new, vulnerable side was quick to speak up.

"I actually don't think I can do that," I'd say.

I feared for my safety attempting a quad in a harness, for example. I didn't trust my body. I didn't believe in my abilities. I was tired of falling and eating the ice. There are only so many spills I could take in a day in my fragile state before it broke me. I hadn't wanted to be truthful before with Frank or Alex or Mitch, because it had been drilled into me that a champion never says, "I can't. It's too hard." But Pasha knew when to push and when to listen, and I came to trust him implicitly. I eventually got to the point where, if he told me to jump, I'd say, "How many times?"

I had to laugh when I finally started showing flashes of the old Gracie, delivering programs that hearkened back to my *Firebird* season, and people questioned why a big-name coach wasn't overseeing my comeback. How sweet of them to think I had had choices.

The truth is, I can count on one hand, with a few fingers left over, the number of coaches willing to take me on when I was fifty pounds overweight and nobody's idea of a meal ticket. I needed people willing to work with the woman I was in my twenties and not compare me to the girl I had been in my teens. Vincent and Pasha and Alex filled that role admirably.

Pasha and Vincent took me out for meals. They sat with me and encouraged me in a nonjudgmental way to eat, which was way harder than it sounds. Losing weight while in recovery from anorexia is a real bitch, and there's not a lot of literature that addresses it, which made me feel like I was the freak in the eating-disorders family. Vincent and Pasha, but especially Pasha, encouraged me to eat normal food in normal portions and let go of the belief that everyone was constantly staring at my plate and silently judging how much or how little food was on it. With their help I gradually grew more comfortable eating in front of other people.

In those early days at IceWorks, I pushed my body for as long as it would allow me. Sometimes it was for only an hour. Sometimes I was able to stay on the ice for multiple sessions. I was having to learn intuitive eating and intuitive skating. In both cases, it required trusting what my body was telling me.

It isn't easy, but if I can put aside my perfectionism for a second, I'm proud of how far I've come since the spring of 2018, when I was still doing cheated double jumps. Most people in the skating world don't have a clue how bad I actually looked on the ice at that point. It was truly pathetic, like watching Michael Phelps if he could only dog-paddle or needed arm floaties.

To be hailed in 2022 as one of the best jumpers in the world in women's skating—by Tara Lipinski, no less—would have been inconceivable in the spring of 2018. To simply land a clean double Axel, which I did without a harness after roughly five months, was thrilling. It's a skill that I'd taken for granted, but relearning it taught me perspective. I read somewhere that less than 6 percent of all skaters have mastered a double Axel. When you start talking about triple Axels, the number shrinks to 1 or 2 percent. For me to expect to land every triple cleanly 100 percent of the time was ridiculous. I was surrounded by people who wouldn't allow me to lose sight of how cool it was that I was doing any of this stuff again.

A big component of my comeback was managing what I could control and letting go of the rest. What people said about me behind my back or on social media or even to my face? Not my problem. I had to picture the words as a balloon and let go of the string. The controllables included upholding my obligations; conducting myself in an honest, honorable way; accepting the outcomes of my actions; acknowledging when I could have done better (and making amends when necessary); and growing every day as a person.

I might have suggested—okay, strongly insinuated—that I was staging a comeback with the Beijing Olympics in my sights. Hey, a girl can dream, right? The 2022 Winter Games were my goal like marrying into the British monarchy could be somebody's goal. It wasn't outside the realm of possibility—I'm looking at you, Meghan Markle!—but so many improbabilities had to click into place, it might as well have been a fairy tale.

Originally, my intent was to return to a level of fitness that would allow me to participate in ice shows. It didn't take much squinting to imagine myself as Elsa in Disney on Ice's production of *Frozen*. But after I landed that first double Axel, my attitude changed. I allowed myself to think, *I've still got it*. I dug my blade a little deeper into the ice. *What if I could compete at nationals again?*

As soon as my coaches saw the shadow of belief flicker across my face, they turned their full powers of persuasion on me: "You can do this. We believe in you. Baby steps." My progress was non-linear, which could be frustrating. As I shed pounds, my center of gravity shifted, which affected the timing of my jumps. As soon as I'd adjust to my new body, I'd lose more weight and have to make more tweaks to my technique. My physical metamorphosis gave rise to mental challenges, walls of doubt that I had to continually push through.

You can't be a skater and have any trepidation about falling; it's a nonstarter, like a fear of heights is for a mountain climber. Over the course of my career, I'd fallen hundreds of thousands of times. I wouldn't say I was used to it, but I had made a bargain with the sport: bruises in exchange for occasional brilliance. But as I began my comeback, my resolve faltered. Every time my ass hit the ice, fear rose in my throat. I was much more attuned to my fragility. I had to build back up my tolerance for falling—for failing—and do it while ignoring the Greek chorus of critics on the sidelines.

Every day I kept showing up. I finally started to gain some momentum in the summer of 2019, when my training became more consistent. There were skaters from my practice sessions whose best days were behind them, but I wasn't one of them. A couple of the teenagers who had been calling me a joke behind my back would soon retire and move on with their lives, as would the teen who told me to my face that I was the rink laughing-stock. I had initially admired her boldness. But now I just skated past her, maybe a tad too close, thinking, *Get out of my way*. I would not be deterred. Every time I stepped on the ice I was hon-oring the memory of the person I credit with saving my life.

17

THE HEARTACHE OF IT ENDING
BEFORE IT EVEN BEGINS

When my phone was returned to me at the end of my stay at The Meadows, I turned it on and steeled myself for the worst. To my relief, it rumbled to life like a Harley-Davidson, loading more emails and texts than I could wade through in a single sitting. More than one of those messages came from John Coughlin.

John was a two-time U.S. national pairs champion from Kansas City, Missouri. I was surprised to hear from him. I would have described us as casual friends, though I had known of him for almost as long as I had been skating. Not long after I had taken my first lessons, John came to Springfield, Missouri, for a skating exhibition. My parents took me and Carly to see it, and I was bowled over. I remember returning home with a fresh resolve, thinking, *So that's what a really, really good skater looks like.*

John was a shepherd who delighted in returning to the flock anyone who was lost. It made him happy to help people. Before the 2017 nationals in Kansas City, I ended up practicing at the same rink as John and his pairs partner. We were the only skaters on the ice and my session didn't go well. It ended with me in tears and with John offering words of encouragement. That was one of the last times we spoke before I got out of rehab.

John was one of the most caring, compassionate people I've ever known. That's how I saw him. Others would view him differently. In their eyes, he was a sexual predator. The disconnect between the person I came to love and the one accused of being a monster by others is something I struggle to make sense of. But I'm getting ahead of myself.

John's first and abiding love was skating. After he retired, he stayed involved in the sport as a commentator, a coach, and an entrepreneur. He was active in the sport's governance through various committees, including the ISU's Athletes Commission.

John's outward cheerfulness hid a deep reservoir of pain. His mother died in 2010 and he endured the disappointment of multiple Olympic qualifying near misses. I used to wish I could roll with adversity as effortlessly as he appeared to. He proved an excellent guide, helping me draw a road map for my post-recovery future.

In our first phone conversation, he asked me if I'd like to team up with him to teach a seminar in Kansas City. As he'd once inspired me in an out-of-the-way rink in Springfield, Missouri, I could galvanize the next generation. But that wasn't his pitch. I'm not sure I'd ever told him about attending one of his exhibitions as a child. No, he presented it as a way for me to make a few bucks and ease my way back into the skating world.

But there was more to it than that. As he confided in Amy, a close friend of his who coached at his home rink and would help us organize and run the clinics, he was concerned about my emotional well-being. He believed I needed to see how beloved I was in the skating community so that I'd have a reason to stick around—in life, not just in skating. In case I was worried (and I was), he wished to put my mind at rest by showing me that my stay in recovery had not rendered me a pariah. My skating family was intact.

I didn't have a good excuse *not* to do it, so off I went down the "Road to Gold," as John named the event. We had a wonderful time. Amy, who was like a surrogate mom to John, was delightful. She said that I must be a strong, brave person to seek treatment for my mental health issues, which was amazing. It hadn't occurred to me that a positive spin could be put on my downward spiral.

That first seminar, and the ones that followed, were magical. It's hard to explain, but the air practically crackled with positive energy. In Kansas City, John and I ended up afterward at a bar that was one of his favorite haunts. We fell into such deep conversation, we completely lost track of time, and I nearly missed my flight home.

I expected our collaboration to be a one-off event. John had other ideas. I kept hearing from him. He'd call and say, *How would you like to teach with me in Bismarck, North Dakota? Birmingham, Alabama?* John and I were patching a hole in skating that I hadn't known existed, seeding the sport in spots that were well off the beaten path. Our act was part vaudeville, part instruction, and total hilarity. Our chemistry was undeniable. Off the ice, it was totally normal for us to start talking and an hour later look at each other and laugh because our conversation had veered so far from the original topic. "How did we get here?" we'd say. The question became one of our inside jokes.

I'm not being dramatic when I say our seminars contributed greatly to my healing. When I was in John's company, I felt more alive. Less alone. We had amazing conversations, but we could also sit in companionable silence. John was brilliant, kind, funny, sarcastic. I never felt more myself than when we were together.

Pretty soon we were talking on the phone every day. John came to my rescue more times than I can count. The money I made from our clinics kept me afloat financially. But his assistance went well beyond that. He was always looking out for me.

When I received an invitation from U.S. Figure Skating to attend the 2018 U.S. Championships in San Jose as a spectator, I was on the fence about going. It would be the last competition before the U.S. Olympic team was finalized—the Olympic team that I had shot all those now useless magazine covers and promos for. I was only a couple of months out of rehab and not sure what kind of reception I could expect. For John, who firmly believed that skating held every answer, there was no question that I would attend. He shut down all of my protestations.

My goal was to blend into the background, but U.S. Figure Skating officials had other ideas. They welcomed me back by leading me to the front row of the VIP section, where, in my paranoia, I could imagine every eyeball in the arena staring at me. Actually, I didn't have to imagine it, and it wasn't paranoia. At one point I glanced up and saw on the giant video scoreboard my face staring back at me. Either an NBC camera or an in-house camera had zoomed in on me at an angle that made me look as round and chinless as Humpty Dumpty. I decided to roll with it. I posted to my Twitter account a screenshot of my boneless face on the giant screen next to a caricature of the moon. Meantime, John swooped in to spirit me away to an unobtrusive seat high in the stands where I could disappear into the crowd.

This would have been the time to pivot to a new passion. It wouldn't have been a stretch to picture myself diving into communications work for NBC or U.S. Figure Skating. As far back as Sochi, I can remember drolly informing the assembled reporters that the beauty of having a journalism degree is you don't have to be a newspaper writer. *Zing!* I wasn't wrong. I envisioned myself riding in helicopters reporting on the traffic—or, because I was living in Los Angeles at the time, a high-speed police chase.

Why didn't I? John had something to do with it. He encouraged me to continue in the sport, but not as an observer. As a participant. He made a persuasive argument: As long as I was capable of competing, why stop? "Walk this path as long as it serves you," he said. On my worst days, it's easy to wonder if I should have stuck to my post-treatment plan to make a clean break from competition, if not from skating. I had scored well on the ACT, so I'm sure some college would have taken me, but I'll never question John's motives. His intentions were pure.

He facilitated my comeback in ways great and small. One time he helped me save face for real. On the way to a competition, I left my makeup bag on the plane. Back when my father was an anesthesiologist in good standing and my sponsors included CoverGirl, it would have been no big deal. I could have replenished my supply with a single phone call or a quick visit to the nearest drugstore. But in 2018 my financial situation was precarious. I was living off my savings and didn't have the disposable income to replace the cosmetics. It was bad enough that I'd already lost my shield of invulnerability. I was terrified of the prospect of competing without my last layer of armor: mascara and lipstick.

I told John what happened, and he explained my predicament to his agent, Tara Modlin, who reached out to her contacts in the cosmetics industry. They responded with loads of makeup that John then overnighted to me.

It wouldn't be the last care package I'd receive from him. That same year, ahead of my twenty-third birthday, he sent me a weighted blanket. When I snuggled under it, I felt the same way I did around John: safe and protected. He enclosed a note with the gift: "Dear Greg: I hope this blanket aids you in your quest of complete solitude." (Greg was one of his nicknames for me. I acquired it when a barista misheard my name during one of our coffee runs and wrote "Greg" on my soy vanilla latte cup.)

John took pleasure in feeling needed and was known for spinning webs of connection. Through him I became friendly with Amy, who has become a surrogate mom to me. He arranged for me to meet his agent, Tara, who now represents me. All you need in life are a few people who believe in you. John and Amy and Tara became those people for me at a time when the distance between me and my family of origin was palpable. Not necessarily for the worse, mind you. I mean, I had to stake my claim to independence at some point.

Not to get all woo-woo, but my bond with John was so intense that I wondered if I had loved him in other lives. My phone archives include a silly video I shot during a clinic we did toward the end of 2018. John and I are sitting in a Birmingham, Alabama, hotel room on adjacent double beds. It's late and John is lying on his back, laughing hysterically at the sound of my voice, which is extra nasally—think Minnie Mouse—because I had spent all day in a cold rink. I don't know what prompted me to press the record button that night. It wasn't like I was capturing him in a rare moment of merriment. John's resting state was joyful. The sound of his laugh was so delightful, like wind chimes in a gale. His laugh made you want to crack a joke just to hear it. I love that video so much. I watch it often. The date stamp is December 30, 2018.

Less than three weeks later, he was gone.

How did we get here? Right before our Alabama trip, the U.S. Center for SafeSport posted on its website that John's eligibility to participate in figure-skating-related activities was being restricted because of unspecified allegations. It was the same organization with which I had lodged a complaint of misconduct against my rapist. Since nothing had come of my filing, part of me worried that this was true for other accusers, too. John's case would swiftly quash that concern.

I appreciate that the burden of proof has to be exceptionally high when a person's freedom is hanging in the balance. As a survivor of a sexual assault, I didn't take the allegations against John lightly. In Birmingham, I waited for him to bring up the matter, and when he did, I could tell that he wasn't confident that things would work out in his favor. He described a deck that was stacked against him. He expressed frustration that he was prohibited in these early stages from telling SafeSport his side of the story, prohibited from addressing the myriad rumors spawned by his inclusion on the organization's website. No charges had been filed. His case was only in the inquiry phase, he said, so why did everybody in skating seem to know and accept as fact the accusations of grooming and sexual misconduct? It was like being questioned for a robbery and at the same time having the conviction show up on your criminal record.

On January 7, 2018, *USA Today* published a story that detailed the allegations against John and included an emailed statement by him:

> While I wish I could speak freely about the unfounded allegations levied against me, SafeSport rules prevent me from doing so since the case remains pending. I note only that the Safe-Sport notice of allegation itself stated that an allegation in no way constitutes a finding by SafeSport or that there is any merit to the allegation.

I had a bad feeling as I read the story. No matter how his case was ultimately decided, it would be hard for him to walk back or live with the awful headlines. I was in regular contact with John during this time. I knew that being ostracized by his skating family was going to devastate him. I knew because when I got out of rehab that had been my fear, too.

Less than a year prior, Larry Nassar, a doctor affiliated with U.S. Gymnastics, had been convicted and sentenced to life imprisonment for grooming and sexually assaulting hundreds of victims over a decades-long span. With U.S. Gymnastics' dereliction of duty fresh in everybody's minds, other national governing bodies were eager to show zero tolerance for predatory behavior. For that, I was grateful. Having recently filed my own report to SafeSport, I was invested in the organization believing the accusers and holding the accused accountable. As an assault survivor, I wanted SafeSport to believe me.

But I also recognized the importance of a full investigation, and John's situation made me see how the system could be corrupted if cases were tried publicly before the facts were fully explored internally. I encouraged John to ride out the investigation.

"If you are able to refute the allegations," I said, "everybody will move on."

"That's where you're wrong," he said. "Even if I prove my innocence, my reputation is ruined."

As the son of a police chief, reputation mattered to John. He always said that popularity comes and goes. Money, too. But the one constant, he said, is character. That core belief had been drilled into him as a child, and now he was being accused of lacking the essence of what made somebody a good human being. In the wake of the allegations, people were quick to distance themselves from John, including some of his closest friends. He had built a post-competition life on connections that he made in skating. If those connections were lost, what would his future look like?

It was a really confusing time. My thoughts were in turmoil. I didn't know how to reconcile the portrait painted of John by his accusers with the person I had come to know and care deeply for. I had to make peace with the fact that all of these things could be true at the same time:

I am a survivor of sexual assault.
John was someone who was there for me at a difficult
      time—my closest confidant.
John might have sexually assaulted women.
Survivors of sexual assault deserve to be believed.
SafeSport didn't act decisively in my case.
It's possible that SafeSport acted too quickly and decisively in
      his case.

Complicating his situation further was that John's physical health was failing. During one of our seminars, I had noticed tremors in his hand. I asked him about it. Parkinson's, he said. He was relatively young to receive such a diagnosis, but he couldn't say he was surprised. His grandparents on both sides had had it. He had lived for years wondering if the same diagnosis awaited him. John said he was seeing a specialist who was monitoring his symptoms.

Let's just say he was far more conversant in the intricacies of health and life insurance plans than any elite athlete in their early thirties should have any reason to be. With any luck, he told me, he'd live to celebrate his fiftieth birthday. He was hopeful but not delusional. He knew that if he was fortunate to still be alive then, he'd probably be wearing a diaper and exhibiting signs of dementia.

In January, weeks after our Birmingham clinic, I pulled out of the upcoming U.S. Championships in Detroit, the competition that was supposed to mark my official return to the national scene. I wasn't ready for that stage, wasn't ready to revisit my memories—most of them awful—of Detroit. On the bright side, with my withdrawal, my schedule opened up. I reached out to John and floated the idea of flying commercially from Philadelphia to Kansas City to keep him company. It was the weekend of January 12. To drive home the point that I was serious, I told him I had already priced some flights.

"Save your money," John told me. He said he was managing fine. "Hold off until you can get a cheaper fare," he said. "We'll catch up then."

Why did I listen to him? I'll never forgive myself for my failure of imagination. I should have pushed back. I knew he was spiraling. But having just come out of my own death spin, I assumed he'd see that, yes, things were shitty and would be for a while, but one day he'd be on the other side of it—just like I was. I was unforgivably blind to the reality of his situation. Because he had saved me, I never thought he would turn around and take his own life. He used to tell me how pissed he'd be if I ever thought of doing such a thing, so why would he leave me behind?

On Thursday, January 17, John was informed by U.S. Figure Skating that he was suspended, not just restricted, from any activities sanctioned by the skating body or the USOPC. He would not be welcome at nationals. He was being excommunicated. Over the next twenty-four hours, I reached out to him numerous times. He never returned my texts.

The next day, Friday, the eighteenth, I accompanied a skating friend named Anthony to a late afternoon matinee of *The Upside* at a Wilmington, Delaware, multiplex near my apartment, which was a fifteen-minute drive from the rink. On my way there, I had a premonition. I called Carly and told her I was worried that John was going to kill himself. She allayed my fears, we hung up, and I ducked inside the theater. For the better part of the next ninety minutes, I laughed until I snorted at the antics of the characters played by Kevin Hart and Bryan Cranston. The comedy provided a welcome break from the emotionally draining events of the past few weeks. I had put my phone on silent and tucked it in my pocket when I sat down, and before the movie was over I could feel it vibrating. I had six missed calls from Carly. That was highly unusual. Also, a text from a Kansas City number that I didn't recognize. *Uh-oh.* Next to me, Anthony's phone was also vibrating. He got out of his seat and took a call from Lisa. I followed him out of the theater and watched as his face clouded over. He looked absolutely stricken, and in that moment, I knew.

Oh no. Anthony was struggling to form words. He was shaking. I told him, "I'm going to call Carly back and she's going to tell me the news. Okay?"

Before I dialed Carly's number, I looked at the text from the 913 area code. Kansas City. It began, "It's Angela. John's sister." I didn't need to read any further. I called Carly, and she delivered the news that John had died by suicide.

He was thirty-three, and as best I can determine he died while I sat in the theater laughing my ass off. I think that John would have appreciated the irony of that. I've wished every day since that he would have hung on until SafeSport finished interviewing witnesses, until the investigation was concluded.

His case was closed after his death, which is unfortunate. The organization's reasoning was that the investigative process exists to protect the sporting community from potential sexual predators, and since John was dead he no longer posed a threat. But without a conclusion to the investigation, there can be no real closure.

In the absence of definitive answers, I carry with me, like rocks in my pockets, weighty questions:

Was I best friends with a predator?
Were other women hurt by someone I dearly loved?
If I miss John, does it make me a monster by proxy?
Why am I still alive and John is not?

These questions still keep me up at night. I loved John deeply and truly. In a parallel universe, I could have imagined us getting married and living happily ever after.

I don't think I'll ever come to grips with his death. I'll live the rest of my life regretting that I didn't follow my instincts and fly out to see him that last weekend he was alive. In my darkest moments, the regret mixes with guilt. He was one of the few people to whom I felt safe exposing my secret self. Did Outofshapeworthlessloser rub off on him and cloud the sunny personality that had managed to burn through my storm clouds?

I've heard that the ending of *The Upside* is hilarious. I'll have to take people's word for it. I'll never be able to finish watching that movie. The multiplex where I received the news of John's death is two miles from my current apartment, but I've never been back. I'll drive miles out of my way to see a movie rather than trigger that memory.

I attended John's funeral in Kansas City. Amy and her husband drove me to the visitation the night prior. When John's sister saw me, she fell into my arms. I got the sense that John had confided in her about how close we had become. "Oh my God, Gracie," she said. "You were the first person I thought of."

There was an open casket at the visitation, which freaked me out. I took one look at the body, turned on my heels, and high-tailed it out of the parking lot. I could not reconcile his waxen face with the person I knew who had been so full of life. His sister tracked me down and stuck an envelope in my hands.

My name was written on the front in John's penmanship. Inside was a letter. I hate to cry in public, but as I read it fat tears rolled down my face:

You mean more to me than you'd probably believe. When I ran into you at nationals and rescued you from the front row where Mitch had stuck you, I felt in that instant that you needed someone to walk with you through the world as you found your feet again. But the truth looking back was that I needed you just as much. You have an uncanny ability to make people smile. My happiest moments this year have been with you on our "work" adventures, but especially the moments spent just bullshitting together in between. I hatched the idea of the clinic in Kansas City partly because I knew it would help you financially, but more because I thought it would be good for your spirit to see just how many girls still looked up to you immensely. Taking our show on the road has become one of my most cherished memories. You know a moment is special when you feel the heartache of it ending before it even begins. And I rested up before each camp because I wanted to be able to stay up for as much time with my best friend as I could soak up. Continue along this path as long as it serves you, and then be fearless as you tackle what's next. You are witty, which means you are brilliant. You are self-deprecating, which means on some level you know just how beautiful you are. You are in-credible to your friends, which means you have it in you to be good to yourself. There's a million things I would do over in life,

but I really think we nailed our friendship. My only regret is
that it didn't last longer. Remember me as the ravioli of a
human that I was. I guess there was some truth to the saying
that the one that laughs hardest carries the most sadness. I love
you to the stars and back.

His "ravioli of a human" line broke me. It was an inside joke
tied to an animated coming-of-age series, *Big Mouth,* that we
both loved. We would recite lines from episodes to each other.
Make what you will of the fact that one of the funniest shows either of us had seen centered around middle schoolers in the
throes of puberty. In the first season, Maya Rudolph, who plays
Connie the Hormone Monstress, called one of the other characters her little ravioli. In his final moments, he paid a sizable but
sad compliment to the show that comforted our angsty souls.

When I finished reading the letter, I called Carly and left a
message, then chain-smoked in the parking lot while I waited for
her to call back. When she finally did, I read the letter to her and
fell to pieces all over again. I've reread it hundreds of times over
the years, and each time I do it's as if John's speaking to me from
the Great Beyond.

After the funeral, a bunch of us ended up at a bar that was one
of John's favorite hangouts to share stories about him and raise a
toast (or several) in his honor. In the days that ensued, I assumed
that Road to Gold would die with John. I couldn't imagine the
seminars continuing on without him. Amy, though, had other
ideas. She saw it as the best possible way to honor his memory.
She made a persuasive argument. Long story short, the seminars
are still going strong.

I was at one in Kansas City, John's hometown, in 2023. Amy
had picked me up at the airport and driven me straight to the
rink. An off-ice session was in progress, and Amy said, "You don't

have to, but would you mind working with the kids on drills?"
"I'd be delighted to," I told her. While I was demonstrating a Lutz
exercise, I landed awkwardly on my left foot and rolled my ankle.
I heard a loud pop. The X-rays confirmed what I already knew. I
had sustained a fracture that would sideline me from skating for
several months. John surely would have appreciated the dark
humor of my competitive career being waylaid in the same city
where my comeback unofficially was launched.

People were taken aback, I'm sure, by the depths of my despair
after John died. Some probably presumed that we must have had
a physical relationship. For the record, we did not. It's almost as if
the connection we had was too sacred to risk ruining it by having
sex. I thought he was my soulmate. I really did. If we were meant
to be together forever, we'd have the rest of our lives to get to
know each other in that way. That he was chaste with me while
possibly violating others is something I'm not sure I'll ever be
able to wrap my head around.

I don't know for sure if John was innocent or not. It's lose-lose
either way. If he was guilty, it means I fell in love with a sexual
predator. What would that make me? His respectability beard?
Or so broken that I gave—and might again give—my heart to the
worst kind of person? It's like a horror movie trope: *The call's
coming from inside the house.* What do I even do with that?

And if he was innocent, the person I fell in love with and
thought I might spend the rest of my life with is dead. He'll live
on in my memories, and in this book. It had to be Chapter 17.
Seventeen was his favorite number. Why? I never asked. All I
know is it held enough meaning to him that he sat for a tat of the
number 17.

I took John's final letter to me and made it the centerpiece of a framed collage that hangs in the main living area of my apartment. Upon walking through my front door, it is the first thing the eye is drawn to. Every time I look at it, I am reminded that everybody is a mystery, even to themselves. And love makes all of us bumbling sleuths.

18

A GOSSAMER THREAD

If I have a free minute, I'll spend an hour browsing Facebook Marketplace, which is where a rustic trestle table caught my eye. The handiwork was exquisite, made even more gorgeous by the twists, swirls, and knots in the walnut. The irregular patterns affirmed my belief that nature really is an artist without peer. I was surprised to learn that the imperfections that I found so fetching were the result of a shock or injury the tree suffered early in its existence that upset its growth.

How I wish I could have afforded that table. Never mind that I had no room for it in my matchbox apartment; I desired the piece for its symbolic value. My post-recovery skating career is like that table. I can't erase the traumas I experienced in my early years; they are a permanent part of me. But I can grow around my imperfections and build something that will be remembered for its beauty.

My comeback has served as an experiment of sorts. Could I be the champion performer that I once was but as a healthier, more vulnerable, person? Would I be able to cleanly land seven triples in a long program if I didn't plow through every practice; if I backed off when I was feeling fatigue or pain or anxiety or light-headedness; if I didn't pretend to be okay when I wasn't?

It's a fine line, a gossamer thread between character-building behaviors and soul-crushing ones. Moments of discomfort are good, up to a point. But where do you draw the line as an athlete, a parent, or a coach? It's a delicate balancing act between pushing myself like I did before, when I'd repeat a failed jump over and over—sometimes as much to punish myself as to get it right—and pulling back because I was veering into mentally unhealthy territory. Between welcoming the physical pain of a practice, because it meant I was getting stronger, and addressing the emotional pain, because my well-being depends on my getting to the root of it.

At eighteen and nineteen and twenty, I was so preoccupied with losing weight and gaining endorsements and changing fourth places into thirds and thirds into firsts, I never soaked up the view from any of the heights I scaled. My eyes were *always* on a bigger summit and a smaller number on the bathroom scale. Post-recovery, I was more grounded. Less unhinged.

Did my skate blades have a little more magic left in them? I couldn't know for sure. But of one thing I was certain: I didn't want to look back in ten or twenty years and wonder what I might have accomplished in the sport if I had only kept going.

I recognized going in that the challenge would be immense. I didn't erase my irregular eating patterns in recovery. I acquired the tools to manage them. What that looked like when I returned to skating—what it still looks like—is a constant, sometimes exhausting bargaining game. Saying no to a chocolate chip cookie or a dinner roll makes me responsible. A good day is when I perceive myself to be smaller than the day before. A better day is when my boyfriend offhandedly remarks that I look fit. The best day is when how I look doesn't matter; when I can quiet the critical voices in my head enough to enjoy a meal out with friends in public. But to manage that I have to research the menu so that I already know what I want to order when I sit down. I've gotten past my calorie-counting days and I no longer weigh myself, but my pre-dining menu routine offers proof that my control issues and anxiety around food aren't totally in the past.

On days when I'm acting really weird about food, I've learned to step back and check in with myself. Am I behaving this way because I'm having a really shit day? Am I using food to regain a sense of control? I'm constantly reminding myself that my thoughts and feelings are valid, but that doesn't mean they're all true. My body dysmorphia is real, sadly, for example, no matter how many people insist that I'm perfect just the way I am or—bless—tell me that I am model thin. As hard as it is for me to manage, it can be downright exasperating to the people who love me. Because what sounds to them like fishing for validation is, in fact, my pleading with them to act as my mirror since I can't trust what I see when I look at my reflection. My grasp of reality is tenuous, at best, when it comes to my physical appearance. It's my biggest mental health issue today and probably will be tomorrow, next year, and two decades from now. I ask the people I trust the most to tell me how I look because I need them to tether me back to reality when I'm spinning. I'm glad I have those people now. They make me wish I'd let others help me when I needed it most.

In July 2018 I received another reality check in the form of the news that Denis Ten, who had been a training mate in Los Angeles, was dead. He had been fatally stabbed by carjackers in his home country, Kazakhstan. Denis had won a bronze in men's singles in Sochi to become Kazakhstan's first figure skating Olympic medalist. He was only twenty-five, younger than I am as I write this.

Denis was a gentle soul who was beloved by everybody at our Los Angeles rink. I knew that he and Frank Carroll were close. I recalled seeing a photo of the two of them that Denis had posted on Instagram less than two weeks before his death. It was obvious what I had to do. Here was a chance to mend a fence.

I waited a couple of days because I didn't want to fire off a pithy "thoughts and prayers" message to Frank in a reflexive response to the tragedy. I took time to craft my words. Frank and I hadn't spoken since our unceremonious split. It was important to me that he recognized my words were coming from a place of genuine caring.

I wrote that I realized our relationship hadn't ended on the most positive note but that I wanted him to know how sorry I was to hear about Denis. He texted me back and thanked me for reaching out. He later said that my gesture showed him that I still cared about him even after all the bullshit we'd been through. I was happy to know that he accepted my text in the spirit in which it was intended, as my apology for everything that had gone down between us.

My relationship with Frank, especially how it ended, is something I regret. We were probably star-crossed from the start. People assume that I must hate Frank because of the messiness of our parting, but I don't. I'm sad at how things ended with both Frank and Alex, but more so Frank, because had the time line been different, I know he would have been my forever coach.

But I had to play the hand I had dealt myself, which meant I was in suburban Philadelphia, not Los Angeles, in the summer of 2018 when I landed the first clean triple Lutz of my comeback during a practice. It was amazing. Everyone at the rink stopped what they were doing and applauded. The joy I felt was genuine. I don't often smile at practice—strike that, I *never* smile at practice—but that day I had an ear-to-ear grin. I had forgotten how magical those moments are, how amazing it feels when you override your overactive mind and find someplace you weren't sure you could go.

I had to make a lot of mental adjustments in those days, most of which centered around accepting that the best version of myself might not ever be the best skater in the world. Or in the United States. Or on the Atlantic seaboard. Wherever I ended up, I had to trust that I would be better off than where I had started. I couldn't lose sight of the big picture. I was showing up every day. That, in itself, represented progress.

Even though I was a two-time national champion, I received no special exemptions into the 2019 nationals. I had to qualify, though there was an express lane open to me. If I participated in a Grand Prix Series event, no matter how I performed, I'd earn a bye into nationals. Otherwise, I'd have to endure two rounds of qualifying. I'm not big on shortcuts, but I had my pride. After competing in the Olympics and multiple world championships and winning two national titles, it would have been a blow to my ego to be relegated to the small rinks and fanfare-free events that I had passed through as a young girl.

So off to Moscow I went for the Rostelecom Cup Grand Prix event in November 2018, accompanied by a reluctant Vincent and by Lisa our rink manager, who was serving as my emotional support person. My coaches weren't wild about the idea. Vincent, in particular, thought it was too soon for me to return to high-level competition. I had only six months of training under my belt, and the emphasis had been on regaining my physical fitness. At this level, so much of the pre-event preparation is geared toward practicing your programs over and over to build up the kind of confidence that will withstand the pressure cooker of competition, which is impossible to replicate in practice. I did not have those repetitions to fall back on, but a transatlantic flight struck me as a better path to nationals than the long road through qualifying.

When Vincent managed to lose his passport in the mail— a ploy by him, I joked at the time, so that he'd have an excuse not to go—I probably should have taken it as an omen. Despite everyone's reservations, I pressed forward. I can be stubborn, and once the idea of competing in Russia had taken root in my head, there was no dislodging it. Looking back, I can see that I was impatient. I had so much ground to make up. My expectations were unreasonable.

My 2014 Olympic teammate Jeremy Abbott choreographed my programs. For the short we'd settled on Annie Lennox's "I Put a Spell on You" after hearing it during one of our car rides. We both loved it, but sadly, I mesmerized absolutely nobody with my performance. I fell on a triple flip, popped my double Axel, and generally labored through the program as if I were skating on sand. I was last in the ten-woman field.

I couldn't imagine subjecting my body, and psyche, to another four minutes and ten seconds of the same. But there is an axiom in skating that you finish what you start. It's one of the aspects of skating that I deeply respect. The battle within the battle; the fight against yourself that, if you can win it, builds confidence and resilience. What life skill is more useful than resilience?

Some of the programs that I am most proud of followed ones that were among my most demoralizing. I didn't want to take the ice for my free skate after my ninth-place short program at the 2013 U.S. Championships, my first at the senior level. But I stayed, landed seven clean triples in my long program, and finished second overall. That's why I generally embrace the philosophy of carrying on.

But as I sat alone in my hotel room in Russia that night after the short program, it struck me as nothing less than an act of masochism to continue. What would I learn about myself that was constructive by performing my free skate? I couldn't come up with a decent answer. I woke up the next morning, shook off a blooming panic attack, and made it to the rink. After a disastrous practice session, I cried on Lisa's shoulder. After talking it over with her, I decided that this was one instance in which surrender was the better part of valor. I withdrew and took to Twitter to explain myself:

I'm heartbroken to withdraw from tonight's free skate. It was a difficult decision to make, but ultimately I need to put my mental health first and focus on the big picture. Looking forward, I need to keep improving both my physical and mental condition. I thought checking into treatment last fall was the most difficult thing I've ever done, but skating my short program last night might have topped it. I do not want to undo the tremendous progress I've made in these last few months and I feel that competing [in] the free skate would be damaging to both my confidence and mental health going into nationals. I thank you all for your support, and I am so sorry if I have let you guys down. This is just the start for me, and I know that greater things are yet to come. Thanks for sticking with me.

To my surprise, the Twitterverse was generally supportive. The social media trolls laid off me, for the most part, and I was heartened by the overwhelming show of compassion. The general consensus among those who reached out to me was that I had scored a triumph of sorts by prioritizing my mental health. One woman thanked me for showing people that it is okay to be broken, which hadn't been my intent. But I had to take my victories where I could find them. *Yay, me!*

If only I could have bottled all that positivity and sipped from it in the weeks that followed. The stench from my performance in Moscow followed me home to Philadelphia, and I just couldn't shake it. Every time I stepped on the ice for a run-through, I got a whiff of failure. If nationals had been anywhere but Detroit, I might have been able to fight through my self-doubts. But in the end, I could not bring myself to return to Michigan when I still felt so shaky. It was too soon. So haunted was I by the memories of my unraveling there, I had rerouted a December trip to California to visit my mother and sister because my original itinerary had me flying through Detroit Metro Airport.

For me, competitions always were more of a mental challenge than a physical one. The phrase people bandied about when talking about me was "basket case." To which I say, you try hurling yourself in the air and completing three revolutions, landing on a sliver of steel, and then throwing yourself back in the air for three more revolutions with the weight of a nation on your shoulders—and your family's happiness hanging in the balance—and then let's talk about being a nervous wreck. I could see where Dorothy Hamill was coming from when she wrote in her 2007 memoir *A Skating Life,* "Competition always felt like I was going to my own execution."

In my case, it too often felt as if I was also the one pulling the trigger.

As soon as I pulled out of nationals, my path back was unavoidable. If I wanted to skate at the 2020 U.S. Championships in

Greensboro, North Carolina, I'd have to advance through regionals and sectionals. It was kind of weird to have fourth-place finishes at the Olympics and the World Championships behind me and local qualifying ahead of me. It's safe to say that I was not fucking stoked to be going back to regionals and sectionals. I thought of Hollywood, which is filled with actors who had to audition after being nominated for or even winning Academy Awards. I remember reading somewhere that Emma Stone was summoned to a casting office to read for a role in the movie *The Favourite* after she had won an Oscar for her leading role in *La La Land.*

And in one of my favorite athlete memoirs, *Open,* Andre Agassi recounted playing in challenger events, several rungs down on the pro tennis ladder, when he was already a three-time Grand Slam men's singles winner (he'd go on to win five more of those, so that challenger stop clearly paid off). If Emma Stone and Andre Agassi could subjugate their egos and get on with the business at hand, so could I. No way did I want my actions to be driven by a fear of failure or the potential for humiliation.

Which is not to say that getting on with it was fun or easy. I'd be interested to know if anyone involved with the casting process asked Emma for a selfie before or after that audition for *The Favourite,* because something similar happened to me. A competitor posed with me at practice and then gushed that I was her idol. To her face, I said, "That's so sweet. Thank you." But I was thinking, *Oh-kay. This is weird.*

I was in uncharted territory, and all I could do was trust the road map that my coaches and I had drawn up. Five days a week, I aimed to complete run-throughs of my programs. On days when I was feeling less than my best—and there were many of those— I redefined progress. Maybe I couldn't finish my free skate, but could I nail a clean triple loop? Before the South Atlantic Regionals, Alex reminded me to skate with freedom and happiness, because no matter where I finished I had already accomplished a lot to get this far.

It wasn't pretty, but I advanced out of regionals, held at IceWorks, with a third-place finish. I knew I had to be much better at the Eastern Sectionals, and I was. At the Hyannis Youth and Community Center in Massachusetts—where the vibes called to mind open-mic night at the corner coffeehouse—I raised my scores above the requirement number on the way to posting another third-place finish. That was good enough to advance to my sixth senior ladies' nationals.

The judges at sectionals had given me high marks for my interpretation of my long program music. No surprise there. I skated to Sara Bareilles's "She Used to Be Mine," and the lyrics struck a hauntingly autobiographical chord for me. The opening line sets the tone: "It's not simple to say, most days I don't recognize me." And then there's the chorus:

She's imperfect but she tries
She is good but she lies
She is hard on herself
She is broken and won't ask for help
She is messy but she's kind
She is lonely most of the time

Behind the scenes, the whole week conjured another Sara Bareilles song: "Gonna Get Over You" ("And I'm not the girl that I intend to be / I dare you, darling, just you wait and see / But this time not for you but just for me"). The Sunday before sectionals, Vincent sent word via text that he would not be able to attend the competition because of personal problems. He actually had the balls to show up at the rink the next day, Monday, and we got into a tragically dramatic screaming fight that started in the IceWorks lobby and spilled into the parking lot. He didn't show up for my Tuesday training session before I left for Massachusetts, and later in the week he just . . . disappeared. Never saw him again. He left behind a note for Alex, who shared a house with him, telling him where he could find the keys to Vincent's leased BMW and asking him to return the car to a dealership in Wilmington, Delaware. He left most of his belongings behind, including framed photographs of his kids atop the living room mantel under his giant-screen TV. None of us have seen or heard from him since, and most of us are still blocked on all of his social media accounts.

It was easily one of the most bizarre things that's ever happened to me, and having gotten this far into the book, dear reader, you know that's saying something. At the time, I had to put my MIA coach out of my mind. I had two months to prepare for nationals, and it was imperative that I improve my jumps and my stamina if I wanted to be competitive.

I was extremely nervous to be back competing on national TV. In my free skate, I singled a planned triple flip in a moment of lost focus that I'd like to think had nothing to do with the Noom ad that I was staring at as I took off. Then again, positioning an ad for an app-based personalized weight-control program, so that it's practically taunting athletes for whom disordered eating is virtually a way of life, is a gold-medal mind fuck.

As a recovering dieter whose eating habits very publicly sabotaged my 2018 Olympic gold medal aspirations, I had a hard time wrapping my head around U.S. Figure Skating's corporate partnership with Noom.

I finished my free skate with my right knee on the ice, my left elbow resting on my bent left knee, and my gaze heavenward, purposefully ignoring the Noom ad in my peripheral vision. The fans stood, and as their applause rained down on me, I teared up. I had sat down earlier in the week with the commentators Tara Lipinski and Johnny Weir, and while I was on the ice Johnny re- called what I had said: "She told us that she felt like she was on a train and she couldn't get off, the way that her whole career was prepackaged, prefab, preprocessed. And she took the power back, she's made all these decisions to come back and it's just so inspir- ing. It takes so much guts to get back under the big lights and this kind of pressure."

I had made Johnny—and the rest of the spectators—feel all the feels, which was a victory in itself. For the first time in my career, I felt as if the crowds had connected with the imperfect person and not the flawless performer Gracie Gold. That's the only ex- planation for why they jumped to their feet for what was objec- tively a so-so performance—three triples, a few downgraded jumps, some strong spins. It was like everyone was celebrating my continued existence. What a powerful feeling. For the first time in my six nationals as a senior, I was fully present as I soaked up the audience reaction. My mind wasn't jumping ahead to the results and what they might hold for my future.

As I waited for my scores, a One Direction song filled the arena: "Right now I'm lookin' at you, and I can't believe / You don't know, oh-oh / You don't know you're beautiful . . ." Now that's what I call a hot take. And speaking of hot takes, it was wild to go back and listen to the commentary provided by Johnny and Tara. Even though I was inarguably less polished than the last time they saw me at nationals in 2017, Tara wasn't questioning my competitive spirit and Johnny wasn't saying I needed to grow up and skate. The word "disastrous" never crossed their lips even though I would finish twelfth, more than seventy points behind the winner, fourteen-year-old Alysa Liu. "So many naysayers, so many people who didn't believe in her," Johnny said. "But she believed in herself." He relayed that I had acknowledged that I wasn't in the best shape of my life but that I was going to try. "And try she did," he said. "Major snaps for Gracie Gold. I can't imagine being in her shoes and coming back . . . Well done, her."

Honestly, I think I liked it better when I was the wounded animal and they were ripping me to pieces like hyenas. I appreciated their acknowledgment of my effort, but a more forthright evaluation of where I was at vis-à-vis the Alysa Lius of the sport would have felt more honest. Could they not evaluate my performance straight down the middle instead of fitting me into a tidy narrative that plays well to the crowd following on TV? In 2016 and 2017 they'd been tearing me down. Now they were building me up as a weepy heroine present to collect my participation trophy—and, indeed, that's how my appearance at subsequent nationals would be framed, as a feel-good story. I never felt as if anybody seriously expected me to be competitive, and after the thrill of my reemergence wore off, that would be reflected in my scores and my press.

I was everybody's choice for Most Inspirational Story and no one's pick to contend. I returned to IceWorks determined to change that.

And then two months later, the whole world stopped.

The ice rink shut down in March, shortly after the coronavirus pandemic was declared, and I was stuck sheltering in place in my two-room apartment. The whole concept of forced seclusion triggered something in me that I thought I had worked through in recovery and therapy.

I wasn't scared of the virus. The isolation is what terrified me. From my time in Detroit, I was painfully aware of what lows I can find when I'm by myself. For someone with a history of using rigid food rituals to cope with a volatile environment and uncomfortable emotions, the loss of my daily physical exercise made me super uptight about gaining back the weight I had shed. I took to staying in bed until noon, because if I was sleeping, I wasn't snacking. All the familiar foods flying off grocery store shelves increased my unease. In my fragile state, the absence of my favorite brand of Greek yogurt could send my anxiety levels skyrocketing. It wasn't as easy as substituting, say, regular yogurt or cottage cheese. I perceived it as a disruption of another essential part of my routine.

The rink's hours remained in flux throughout the fall, reopening and closing as local public safety mandates dictated. I spent months in a state of high alert. We all became like passengers at the gate of a commercial flight delayed by factors out of the control of the people in charge, who ordered us to board, then deplane, board, then deplane, as the information at their disposal changed. All that energy was being wasted to get nowhere. When we were permitted in the building, I'd spend hours upon hours on the ice, as if I could make up for a month of lost training sessions in a single week. I was panicked about staying in shape and not gaining weight, which are two separate issues. I lacked the perspective to step back and see the big picture. Given the toll the pandemic was taking on so many people—the lives and livelihoods lost or forever altered—it wasn't the end of the world if my progress stalled. In the grand scheme of things, I was well ahead of the game even if my skating went backward. If ever there was a time to give myself a break, it was now.

Instead, I doubled down. My attitude was *I need to do more. I need to push through whatever discomfort I'm feeling.* In the summer of 2020, I totally overdid it. If there was available ice time, I took it and made use of every last second. I turned twenty-five in August. No matter what music I was skating to, my soundtrack was my ticking physiological clock. I was already old for a figure skater, and I had miles to go to be competitive again. And so I pushed myself too hard. I wore out my boots, wore out my blades, wore out my body. By the start of the fall, I was experiencing pain caused by an alignment issue in my right hip.

I was in a shambles mentally and physically by the time I took part in a Skate America event in October 2020. I received the worst overall scores of my eight years in senior competition to place last in the twelve-woman field. And let me tell you, those shitty scores were deserved.

I had no time for a pity party because in December I had to submit a video of a proctored free skate that would be scored by a panel of judges. There were forty-six entries. The top nine earned berths to the nationals in Las Vegas, Nevada. I finished seventh to qualify for my seventh senior-level nationals.

It was a lost cause. I finished thirteenth at nationals, one spot lower than the year before. I felt deflated. The Beijing Olympics were one year away. Instead of being hopeful that anything could happen between now and then, I worried that my window for being competitive was not just closed but had been nailed shut.

I was not in a good headspace when I reached out to Carly to vent. She had heard enough. She texted me back and said:

The whole world is just emerging from a year-long pandemic. What did you expect, business as usual? Give yourself a break. You embarked on this comeback for the love of the sport and so you could finish your career on your own terms. If you aren't loving it, if you're done with it, just retire already. But don't stay in the sport and make yourself and everyone around you miserable.

Carly was right, even if I didn't enjoy hearing it. She knows me better than I know myself. I was wearing out everybody who cared about me.

And then, miraculously, I found someone new to love—and to lean on.

19

BUILDING MY NEST

I'll be making a list, a program of tasks to be completed in a certain sequence to ensure that my day runs smoothly, and I'll lose track of time. The next thing I know, an hour has passed and I have an interview that was scheduled to start one minute ago and less than five minutes to move my parked car before it's ticketed. As I'm flying around the apartment, upending articles of clothing and cushions in search of my keys and texting the person awaiting my call on my cellphone to let them know I'm running late, I have to shush Outofshapeworthlessloser, who is saying for the umpteenth time, *Why can't you be different? Just be better* is a refrain that floats around in my head like an algae bloom.

Skating offers me the perfect cover. It's a safe place to hide my personality quirks. I was diagnosed in my twenties with attention deficit hyperactivity disorder, and I'm on medication for it. The more I learn about it, the more aha moments I have. It places into context why I'm likely to fall behind or forget or lose the thread completely with maddening regularity. I believe my ADHD holds the answer for why I tend to let tasks accumulate until I'm buried under an avalanche of incomplete chores and outstanding obligations.

What I need is a Lori Nichol or Jeremy Abbott to choreograph my life.

A memory resurfaces: I am in grade school, fourth grade maybe, and I have a writing assignment. I can't remember what the subject was, but I do recall having big ideas that I poured out on page after page after page. I vividly recall Mom looking at it and lecturing me. It wasn't bad, she said, but I wasn't a very good editor. *No teacher has time to read twelve pages, Gracie.* Her subtext seemed clear: I needed to be more organized in my thoughts and deeds.

I used to be bothered by my brain wiring, which drops these issues in my lap like a knotted skein of yarn and says, *Here, you untangle this.* It probably goes without saying that a teenager flying to the Olympics cuddling her baby blanket might scream neurodivergent. So might a grown woman who has to be cajoled by her boyfriend to wear something more becoming than oversized sweats to eat out at a nice restaurant because the seams in most articles of clothing are excruciating on her skin. I wish sometimes that it weren't so, but this is me in my many-splendored messiness.

In the past I'd have given anything to be easygoing. Chill. But I'm not. I can be difficult. Oddly enough, I've recently grown to like my personality. *I am who I am.* That said, I'm aware that I evoke strong reactions in people. They either love me or cannot stand me. Given that my job is to please nine judges and thousands of spectators and a television audience in the millions, a polarizing personality can feel like a curse.

I used to carry around my evil eye key chain to ward off the bane that is my brain. But then I heard a story about a mango during a therapy session, and it made all the difference in how I see myself. Imagine, my psychologist said, that you are the most beautifully colored, luscious, ripe, flavorful, superior-grade mango that ever was plucked from a tree. You could be a mango larger and lovelier and more delicious than any other elsewhere in the world and it won't matter to some people. To those who don't like the taste of mangoes or are put off by their texture, you will be rejected outright for no reason other than mangoes aren't their jam.

My job, she said, is to find the mango lovers.

For someone trained to please others on the ice, the mango story was life-changing. I had spent most of my first twenty-two years trying as hard as I could to win over people who were never going to like me because I simply wasn't their piece of fruit.

Post-recovery, I've become intentional about the company I keep. I surround myself with people who won't be turned off by my difficulties managing appointments, emotions, impulses, paragraphs, schedules. People who won't stop me if I'm rambling too long or make me feel embarrassed or ashamed, as if whatever I was saying was boring or unimportant. I want to be around people who will challenge me to become the best version of myself as opposed to someone entirely different. I've learned that good people can be found in the unlikeliest places, such as a worn rink in suburban Philadelphia that, like me, has seen better days.

Out went the vultures feeding on my carcass, cast aside to make room in my nest for kinder birds who nourish me. I'm a firm believer that people come into your life at the precise moment you need them. Their importance in your life is not to be measured in how long they exist on your time line but how genuine and impactful their presence is in their time with you.

Spring 2021, the season of rebirth. An ice dancer at IceWorks caught my eye. His name was James Hernandez, and he was back in the States after riding out the pandemic in his native Britain. I was tempted to look away when I discovered he was six years younger than I am. Age boundaries get blurred all the time in skating because athletes are lumped together by ability, making it commonplace for teenagers to be mingling with those in their twenties. But outside skating, I worried that my attraction to James could be perceived as weird. The double standard wasn't lost on me. My father had affairs with women a decade or two younger than him and nobody blinked. But a twenty-five-year-old woman attracted to a nineteen-year-old man? I could hear the Greek chorus chanting, *Cradle-robber.* Oh, wait. That chorus was two men who were regulars at my rink.

If James and I had met ten or twenty years from now, our age difference would have set no tongues wagging and zero eyebrows arching. But in 2021, it felt . . . complicated. What could be more on-brand for me? Why pursue a run-of-the-mill romance when an extreme version existed? If you met James, you'd understand why I cast aside my reservations and chose to take the leap. He is an empathetic and sweet man who bears more than a passing resemblance to the English actor Hugh Dancy. And when he opens his mouth to speak, his British accent is bloody brilliant at holding my attention.

James and I got to know each other better as IceWorks prepared for its 2021 show. I choreographed a number and so did he. When his skaters were on the ice, I made a point of casually leaning in to him. "You worked on this one, right?" I cooed.

The physical contact did not have its desired effect. Yes, he said, and turned his attention back to the ice. Undeterred, I engaged with my wingman, another coach at the rink whom I could count on to have my back. He oversaw the coaching roster for the group lesson program at IceWorks, and since James, like me, was also instructing on the side, I asked him to kindly schedule us for the same classes. And still the poor dear was oblivious to my affections. Bless him, he thought it was a crazy coincidence that we left the rink at the same time night after night.

His cluelessness only enhanced his appeal. On our way out the door of the rink at the end of the day, I'd engage him in small talk. Pretty soon we were conversing for an hour or more next to our cars until we were the only ones left in the parking lot.

I shot my shot. Apparently none too subtly. The other skaters observed this awkward dance and started pestering me. They wanted to know if James and I had gone out yet. My interest in him was painfully obvious to everyone. Except him.

What was my next move? I had no idea. James was billeting with a family at the time, and when he casually mentioned our parking lot conversations to his female host and said he thought I might be hitting on him, she laughed out loud. *I'm sure you're mistaken,* she said. *She's probably just being nice.* Our relationship might have been sunk before it ever left the dock if it hadn't been for someone finally coming right out and saying, *James, Gracie is into you.*

Long story short, that's how we ended up meeting for coffee on what I consider our first date. We had several more of these coffee dates over the next two months before James realized we were going out.

Eventually, James moved in with me. He does most of the cooking, the only exception being anything that requires marinating because his idea of seasoning is HP Sauce. Having someone take over mealtimes has been a big benefit to me. It means I can no longer get by living off coffee and cigarettes and a daily tomato. He leaves me with no excuse not to eat at least one healthy meal a day. He's sympathetic to my food anxieties, which is why he takes a black Sharpie and draws a line through the calorie counts on every food label from the store before he puts the items away in our refrigerator or cupboards.

I do my best to nourish him, too. He struggles with self-belief, not so much as a performer but as a person. He is a classic "pleaser," and people often abuse his kindness and generosity, so I'm teaching him how to be a bitch when necessary. I'm forever reminding him that it's fine to be the villain in somebody else's story if that's what it takes to protect his own peace. I am also constantly reiterating something that is hard for us judged athletes to grasp: How other people feel about him is none of his business.

The most challenging thing for us has been to learn how to fight because we both have big feelings that we bottle up, though for different reasons. For James, it's to protect other people, and for me, it's an act of self-defense. On the rare occasions when those big feelings get uncorked, James's tendency is to trail after me, hammering home whatever point he's trying to make to win the argument, which is triggering to me because it's reminiscent of every fight I had with my mom growing up. Then, I tended to stubbornly stand my ground, refusing to back down.

With James, I've made great strides in de-escalating conflict in general. I'll tell him that I need five minutes alone to gather myself. I'll go into the bathroom, sit on the toilet, and let my nervous system calm down while I play over in my mind how a seemingly mild conversation went off the rails. Or I'll say that I need to get something out of the car or move the car and that I'll be back in five minutes, and I'll go sit behind the wheel without starting the ignition and decompress. On occasion I'll text Carly, give her a synopsis of the argument, and ask her if I need to apologize. More times than not, after replaying the fight in my mind or consulting with Carly, I'll emerge from the bathroom or my car and tell James I'm sorry, I'll explain why what he said made me reactive, and we'll end up laughing with (not at) each other.

Given our tendency to suppress our anger, I thought it would be fun for James's birthday one year to give him a couple's rage room visit. Nothing says I love you like shattered fine English bone china teacups. We happily spent half an hour destroying glass, porcelain, and wood objects using sledgehammers and baseball bats. All I can say is it was *extremely* therapeutic. As I was taking the sledgehammer back, it occurred to me that they really ought to have a rage room next to the kiss-and-cry area at competitions. Now *that* would be just what the psychologist ordered after a bad program.

On our first anniversary, I gave James a personalized painting that I had done. I sent my favorite photograph of us to a company that sent me back a canvas with paint-by-number color instructions. It took me a while to finish it, but even I couldn't find fault with the result. The painting really does look like the photograph. That was the second big gift I gave him. The first one was actually a present that we gave each other.

In October 2021, roughly three months before the U.S. Championships in Nashville, Tennessee, we acquired a high-maintenance pet, a fur baby named Teddy who is considered a unicorn in the cat world. Teddy is a caramel-and-white Scottish Kilt, a cross between a Scottish Fold and a Munchkin. He has the folded ears of the Scottish Fold, a breed I've adored since Taylor Swift posted photographs of hers, and the short legs of the Munchkin.

My initial idea was to foster a pet, but a deep dive online led me to a litter of Scottish Kilt kittens for sale in Scranton, Pennsylvania, a two-hour drive from the rink. One day after we were done skating, James and I made the commute to check out the litter. Teddy was the only kitten left. He had short legs, which is what I thought was so cute about him at the time, only to realize with a start later that those short legs that I found so adorable are a deformity that will potentially cause him myriad issues and discomfort later in his life.

This breaks my heart because I've loved him from the instant we met.

So eager was the owner to unload him, I got Teddy for a song. The mama cat mewled loudly as we were leaving, which sent James into spasmodic sobbing. "We took him from his mum! We took her baby!" he wailed.

We sat in the car for several minutes until he calmed down. James, that is. Teddy was chill.

Teddy was maybe four pounds when we brought him home. Over the next several days we thought he might be experiencing separation anxiety from his mom, because he wasn't eating or drinking. Naturally, his issues with eating made me love him only more. He was diagnosed with anorexia (like mother, like fur baby), at which point James and I started bottle-feeding him water mixed with supplements and hand-feeding him a special kind of kitten gel.

Teddy wasn't thriving, but we slowly started to bond—at least when I could find him. My prewar apartment has parquet floors and Teddy blended into them so well that sometimes I thought I'd lost him. I called James once in a panic, fearful that perhaps Teddy had snuck out the door when I wasn't paying attention. It turned out he was curled in a ball under the couch. I had looked there but my eyes hadn't registered him.

At his first vet appointment, the receptionist at the front desk brightened when we walked through the door.

"Hi, are you our two o'clock?" she said. "We've been waiting for you!"

James nudged me and whispered, "Oh my God, Gracie, they know who you are!"

It was sweet of him to think that, but also impossible since the appointment was under his name. In fact, Teddy was the star. The confirmation came when *multiple* vet assistants swooned and said, "Oh, a Scottish Kilt! We don't see these very often."

Teddy turned out to be a very sick kitty. The first three vets we took him to had no fucking idea what was wrong with him. The third vet visit was to a twenty-four-hour animal hospital where James and I spent our first New Year's Eve as a couple together (so romantic—not). There it was recommended that we take Teddy to an East Coast specialist named Dr. F. We did, and Dr. F. was the one who diagnosed Teddy with feline infectious peritonitis (FIP). Perhaps nothing screams Gracie Gold more than my having a cat with eating issues that require a vet neurologist.

Full disclosure: I wouldn't trade Teddy for the world. I love him to pieces, but having since educated myself about his breed, I will never again purchase a "designer" cat because of the "cute" deformities that can be, in fact, debilitating, and I'll also avoid the careless backyard breeders who risk the welfare of the animals under their care when they don't adequately address all the needs of the mother and her offspring. It was irresponsible of me, and I want the pet lovers of the world to know that I have learned my lesson and promise to do better moving forward.

The medication to treat Teddy's disease had not been FDA-approved. As I understand it, it wasn't because the treatment was ineffective but because of concerns that the human population would snatch up the supply for its own use, as happened with ivermectin, a medicine commonly used to treat worms in large animals like horses. I was advised to sign up with an FIP Warriors Facebook group, and through that avenue, I gained access to a treatment known as GS-441524.

It was not cheap. It cost thousands of dollars a month for eighty-four consecutive daily injections. It was not money that I could access by slipping my debit card into the nearest ATM. A generous friend offered to put the cost on their credit card and let us pay them back in monthly installments.

Nor was the medicine for the faint of heart, since it was injected with a syringe and a needle. Which was dramatic, since I hate needles. Every time I stuck that golden serum in Teddy's skin, it didn't escape me that I was going to all this time, trouble, and expense to save Teddy when not that long ago I had been ambivalent about keeping myself alive. Sounds bizarre, right? Actually, it makes sense. When you're struggling with your mental health, it can be exhausting to look after yourself. But if you have pets or people dependent on you for their survival, keeping them alive can be a powerful catalyst for your own continued existence.

Teddy requires us to rise early to feed him, which tethers me to the here and now. I can't dismiss his care as easily as I can my own. I might blow off the meditative exercises that calm my mind, but I'm diligent about turning on Cat TV for Teddy on my way out the door so he can be soothed by the sounds of nature and spa-like music while James and I are both gone.

It's the paradox of poor mental health: You can be loving to others even when struggling with self-loathing. Ultimately, the act of reaching out to others is how I rescue myself. When I isolate myself, despair rushes in to keep my depression company. The first couple of days of Teddy's treatment were traumatic for us. Teddy didn't seem to care much for them, either. During one of the injections, Teddy clawed me on the right arm and left gashes that looked just like the slits people intent on self-harm make on their wrists and lower arms. Thank God I love long-sleeved turtlenecks, because I lived in them until the scratch marks healed.

I entertained some seriously dark thoughts that I was to blame for Teddy's poor health. Had I done something to expose him to the virus? Had I arranged for his second round of vaccines too early? Eventually, I let it go. The probabilities are that his mom was infected and transmitted it to Teddy before we laid eyes on him. But it's all immaterial. All that mattered was that James and I did everything in our power to help him.

Poor James. Teddy was still at death's door when I had to leave my two boys for the 2022 nationals. The timing couldn't have been worse. James was spending as much time in Dr. F.'s office as he was at IceWorks. James wanted to travel to Nashville to cheer me on, but the obstacles in his path seemed insurmountable. The cost, for one. But mostly: How could he leave Teddy with his health so precarious? In desperation, James called Dr. F. He explained that we both had to go out of town. Was there any way he could watch Teddy? It was a big ask, but Dr. F. didn't blink. "I'd be happy to," he said.

There's a funny postscript. Dr. F. knew me only as Teddy's mom. The day after my short program, which was televised, James received a sheepish text from him: "I think I've put two and two together. You're in Nashville, right?"

My cover was blown. All thanks to Teddy—who's doing fabulously, by the way. He's living his best life. James, too. As for me, I can't complain. Every time James and I dine at our favorite neighborhood restaurant, Del Pez, we order blended mango margaritas and clink our glasses in a toast: "To us." Those margaritas are one of our favorite (and most delicious) inside jokes.

20

EAST OF EDEN

It was not a given that we'd skate in front of fans in Nashville at the 2022 U.S. Championships. The U.S. Olympic speedskating trials, held in Wisconsin at roughly the same time, took place behind closed doors because of a surge in COVID-19 cases, and U.S. Figure Skating officials seriously considered having us skate in an empty Bridgestone Arena to better protect us from becoming infected with the omicron variant.

After much discussion, the call was made to allow spectators who could show proof of a COVID-19 vaccination, and to test competitors before and during the competition. That decision made possible one of the most meaningful moments of my career. For my short program, I chose to skate to *East of Eden*, an orchestral piece that my childhood idol, Michelle Kwan, had memorably performed to during her career.

I'd wanted to *be* Michelle since early in my skating career. The closest I came wasn't even on the ice. It was during Spirit Week one year in middle school and we were encouraged to dress up as our idols. Mom being Mom, she went all out to transform me into a mini-Michelle. I wore a red dress with a big Chinese gold dragon on the front. We spray-dyed my hair black and I wore big-winged eyeliner that extended almost out to my temples. Looking back, I can see how uncool it was to appropriate someone else's culture. But my love for Michelle ran so deep, I honestly thought wanting to be exactly like her was the best compliment I could pay her.

I was dressed like myself the first time I met her. It was backstage at an ice show, and in my excitement, I neglected to bring a program or piece of paper for her to autograph. When I got to the front of the line, I whipped off my dirty sneaker and handed it to her to sign. It mortified my mom but didn't faze Michelle at all. She signed my shoe without hesitation.

I admire Michelle so much for the way she remained at the top of her game for more than a decade, ignoring all the people who told her that it was time to move on and disregarding those who'd have her believe that the only measure of success was an Olympic gold medal.

Michelle was everything I wasn't. She was reliable and consistent at events. She skated with her heart on her sleeve and connected with the audience every single performance. She was the ideal student and hung on Frank Carroll's every word (until she abruptly parted ways with him four months ahead of the 2002 Olympics).

Having Frank as my coach and performing to her signature music was as near as I'd ever come to mirroring her legendary career. I had expressed for several years the desire to perform to *East of Eden* but had always been dissuaded from doing so. Because Michelle had embodied the piece so beautifully, other skaters couldn't help but suffer in comparison.

East of Eden was another of my declarations of independence. I was determined to skate to it and nobody could stop me. Whatever happened in Nashville, I would own it. My program. My choice. The day of the women's short program, I started my morning in normal event-day fashion. I called Carly and Mom and sobbed to the point of dry heaving about everything that could go wrong.

Funnily enough, after all the hand-wringing over whether or not to welcome a ticket-buying audience, it looked for a while as if we might be skating in an empty arena anyway. An overnight blizzard dumped so much snow and ice on the roads, travel to the arena was treacherous. Mom and Carly were staying in a short-term rental two miles away and couldn't maneuver their cheap rental car out of the driveway because of the ice. Plan B was to use a rideshare app, but when one driver after another canceled on them because of the hazardous road conditions, they resorted to Plan C. They hoofed it the two miles, powering through snowdrifts in their sneakers as Carly sang "Do You Hear the People Sing?" from the *Les Misérables* soundtrack to tamp down her anxiety about being late.

James also cut it close. He traveled from Philadelphia by plane the day of the short, and the bad weather caused his flight to be delayed. His plane landed in Nashville less than an hour before I was scheduled to leave my hotel for the arena. He couldn't find a cab or rideshare, but my golden-retriever boyfriend's gregarious personality saved the day (as it often does). He had made friends during the flight with a mother and her son, and they offered to give him a lift downtown. From where they dropped him off, he walked the last few blocks to my hotel. We left for the arena together, and Carly and Mom joined him in their nosebleed seats right before I took the ice.

Upon being introduced, you have thirty seconds to position yourself at center ice. That does and doesn't feel like an eternity. In those thirty seconds, I usually have one technical thought that

I'm repeating almost as a mantra. In Nashville, a lot was going through my mind. This was basically my Olympic moment, my one chance to make *East of Eden* my own and show the judges what I'd been showing Pasha and Alex every day in training.

The music began, and my muscle memory took over. My opening combination was a triple Lutz–triple toe, which I landed.

In the stands, Mom, Carly, and James heaved a collective sigh of relief. They understood how critical it was for the rest of my program that I hit those two jumps. I slightly underrotated the triple toe, but whatever. I remained upright.

One minute into the program came my double Axel. You know how the Hall of Fame basketball player Shaquille O'Neal struggled with free throws? For his NBA career, he shot 58 percent with hands in his face and big bodies in his space. And *53 percent* from the foul line with nobody contesting his shot. What free throws were to Shaq, the double Axel was to me. If there was a jump that I consistently missed in competitions, it was the double Axel, the only jump that takes off forward. You launch from a forward outside edge and complete two and a half revolutions in the air before landing on the back outside edge of the opposite skate. It's a polarizing jump. Skaters either hate it or love it. I loved it. The problem was, it hated me. Over the years, I received all kinds of advice about how to nail it. It used to kill me. Did people think I didn't practice the double Axel every damn day? I would consistently complete the jump with air to spare in practice. But under intense pressure, all bets were off. I couldn't afford a shitty double Axel, and because I was aiming for perfection, my mind would freeze, and I'd either open up and pop to a single Axel or rush the double and wind up on my ass.

Every time I missed the jump in competition, I became exponentially more nervous about performing it the next time. Landing it turned into psychological warfare. Thankfully, Pasha and

Alex helped me reset my double Axel so that it became much more reliable, to the point where people commented on how big a jump it had become for me.

In my short program in Nashville, I nailed it and my face lit up. You can see me beaming in the video on YouTube.

As soon as I lifted off for my last big element, a triple loop, I knew the jump was money. The rest of the way, I concentrated on softening my arms and knees and carving clean turns. I fought my tendency, when tired or tense, to look more like an automaton than an ice princess. I went into my last spin thinking, *Don't fuck it up now.*

After the final note of my music, I was almost lifted off my feet by a tsunami of sound. The fans had stood and were cheering and clapping. It took me a second to read the arena. I was confused. I hadn't been flawless, so why was I getting this standing ovation? And then it hit me. I had pulled the fans out of their seats. Me.

I had connected to the music and to the crowd. In an age of wonder kids jumping out of their skates to produce athletically admirable but emotionally empty highlight reels, my mature performance struck a chord. People were moved by it. My hands flew to my face. I'm an ugly crier, which is why I am a public stoic, but I didn't even attempt to blink away the tears welling in my eyes.

I can count on one hand the number of times in my career that I delivered a performance that burrowed into people's hearts. It delighted me to start so strongly, and at a nationals to boot. It's always a tricky event because the atmosphere is supercharged. I was extra proud of myself because I'd basically had to relearn every element in that two-minute-and-fifty-second program. Given my tragic track record in short programs at nationals, nailing this one felt really satisfying. And the standing ovation is something I'll carry with me the rest of my life. When I met with reporters afterward, I said, "I really did everything that you could want. To nail almost everything. Not perfect-perfect, but what can you want?"

I had held my nerve. Not just that. For the first time in years—I don't know, maybe *ever*—I hadn't performed my program. I had *become* it. I had told a story using my body. I felt good bordering on giddy.

My score was 67.61. A smidge low, I thought. Gone were the days when judges would give me strong program component (also known as artistic) marks or better grades of execution on my elements even if my skating hadn't been my best. I had squandered their goodwill with a year of lackluster programs, followed by forty-five days in a recovery center. Not until I lost my special treatment did I fully appreciate the extent to which the sport is set up to maintain the status quo. No matter. My score was thirteen points higher than my short program scores at the prior two nationals and my best short program total since the 2016 World Championships. It put me in sixth place, which secured me a spot in the final group for the free skate. Not bad considering I had to advance through regionals and sectionals to earn my spot in the field.

Besides which, the judges weren't *really* the ones I had been skating for. When I finally met up with James, I asked, "Was it good?" James is a perfectionist like me. He's not one to dole out praise indiscriminately. I knew I could count on him not to blow smoke up my ass. There were plenty of days in training when I'd ask him to critique my triple Lutz and he'd shrug and say, "Maybe it's not a Lutz day."

But this time he said, "It was fucking amazing!"

My night was made.

It got better. James and my agent, Tara, scrolled through social media and shared with me some of the comments about my program. This one was sweet: "You brought this grumpy, pugnacious, 61-year-old man to tears. I will NEVER forget that performance for the rest of my cynical life."

But my hands-down favorite came from Jen Psaki, President Biden's badass press secretary, who tweeted, *Gracie Gold tonight after everything she's been through is an incredible story.*

As James and I made the ten-minute walk from the arena to the hotel, the stillness of the night was broken by the cries of passersby.

"I love you, Gracie!"

"Good luck tomorrow, Gracie!"

It was magical.

If only the story of my 2022 U.S. Championships had ended there.

21

"THERE'S AN OLYMPIC SPOT FOR GRACIE GOLD!"

Some people prefer the short program because of its brevity. But the less that is asked of you, the more minuscule the margin for error. One mistake and you can kiss that straight-A goodbye. I had built a whole career of coming back after poor shorts at nationals, but after such a solid start in Nashville, I could go into the free skate feeling none of the usual pressure to be flawless because I was essentially skating with what amounted to house money. Right?

I wish.

By the time I arrived at the rink, my podium prospects had improved. Alysa Liu, who was three spots ahead of me, withdrew after testing positive for COVID-19, moving me up to fifth. She was one of a handful of athletes to be infected with the virus that week, which activated a contact-tracing process that served as a stressful reminder that any of the rest of us could be next. One of the skaters ahead of me, Isabeau Levito, was fourteen, which made her too young to qualify for the Olympics if not the podium. I essentially stood in fourth place—my favorite spot (ha ha)—with three Olympic berths on offer. The actual math was more complicated, because Alysa could be put on the team based on her overall season results, and I hadn't achieved an Olympic qualifying score in international competition. But figure skating, with its subjective judging and internecine politics, has never been particularly bothered by objective facts.

I had succeeded in the short program by focusing on the process. Beijing had been a dot on a distant horizon. But suddenly I couldn't round a corner in the arena without hearing the O-word. *There's an Olympic spot for Gracie Gold! There's an Olympic spot for Gracie Gold! There's an Olympic spot for Gracie Gold! There's an Olympic spot for Gracie Gold! There's an Olympic spot for Gracie Gold!* In less than twenty-four hours the conversation had shifted from how far I'd come to how close I was to staking a legitimate claim to a U.S. Olympic berth.

I wish I could say I turned up Noah Kahan in my earbuds and drowned out the outside noise. But the chatter inside my head was the problem. In an instant, my perspective had changed and so had my focus. Paralysis by overanalysis set in. It was as if I had been journaling for catharsis these last five years and overnight I became aware that my words would be published. My stress levels spiked. My fear and dread that I might let people down became acute.

A clean free skate and I'd give those in charge of finalizing the Olympic team cause to pause. A clean free skate and I'd make the podium at nationals for the first time since 2016. Those were big carrots and until then my goals had been small: stay in the moment, soak up the experience. I had arrived in Nashville with no Olympic expectations, no delusions that I deserved to be in the mix of U.S. candidates. My comeback had been built on letting go of the Gracie Gold who was the face of U.S. women's figure skating and embracing who and where I was at this moment in time. All the talk about the Olympics took me back to that time before my mental health crisis when my face was splashed on all the event programs and the posters and the expectations were huge. My body responded in kind, with physiological changes that were palpable. My breath grew shallower. My heart was beating so fast, I thought I was going to faint.

I asked Pasha and Alex, "Are people expecting me to go out and win tonight?"

I asked James, "What if I don't do it?"

They did their best to redirect my thoughts, but it was too late. I was in full freak-out mode.

My choice of music for the free skate was *Daphnis et Chloé,* an orchestral piece that I had used during the 2016–17 season. *Daphnis et Chloé* had not been my undoing then. It was not the reason I performed so poorly. The music was the vanilla pudding that you eat before you become violently ill with a stomach virus. The vanilla pudding isn't what made you sick, but you can't ever eat it again because of its association with the extremely unpleasant memory of throwing up all over yourself.

Daphnis et Chloé was such a gorgeous piece. I wanted to purge it of all the bad memories that I associated with it. My friend and fellow Olympian Jeremy Abbott had touched up the choreography, and I really liked it. Different look, same rough result. The best thing I can say is that I didn't go splat. I touched my hand on the ice on my opening triple Lutz, which I was meant to follow with a triple toe loop. But I bailed on the second triple and it went downhill from there. I stumbled out of a triple flip, doubled a triple Salchow, doubled a triple toe loop.

I never stopped fighting, but I was battling myself the entire four minutes and ten seconds. I had to lean on all my years of training to continue smiling, to convey through my facial expressions that it was a supreme honor to be on the ice making a fool of myself. The mask mandates were in place, mercifully, so I was able to hide my despair somewhat after I was done, though I broke down in tears in the kiss-and-cry area while hugging a giant teddy bear.

I finished twelfth in the free skate, tenth overall. My mom and sister didn't bother to stay until the end. They left the building as soon as I was done. They knew it was fruitless to try talking to me. Poor James. To him fell the unpleasant task of escorting me back to the hotel. We walked in silence. In contrast to the night before, I heard not a single *I love you, Gracie!* Except from James, which was lovely.

Back at the hotel, I blocked anyone who reached out to me by email or text and began with, *I know you're disappointed in your finish, but . . .* I had no patience for people stating the obvious. There were no buts about it. It was not a wonderful week. I was claiming no moral victories. I was so down, I snarled at Carly for saying "Keep your chin up."

I know. Dramatic, much? But hear me out. Can't people simply acknowledge my pain? Why does everybody feel compelled to try to erase it and, in effect, erase me? See me. Please. The end of every dream, every season, every Olympic cycle, every career—these are all mini-deaths to be mourned. It is not a time for toxic positivity, for upbeat messages about how I should be happy it happened instead of sorry it's over. I know my big feelings are uncomfortable, but they are part of me. Dismiss them and you are essentially rejecting me.

It is not helpful to say, "I hope you don't feel sad." Too late. I'm already there. And for fuck's sake, don't tell me, "You tried really hard." Do you think I want to be reminded that that shit program was the best I was capable of?

Nor do I want to hear that I'm "amazing." You might think you're lifting me up, but you're not. You're making me feel as if what I'm experiencing is not the "correct" emotion. It pisses me off to have my feelings invalidated.

Approach me with soothing noises and I'm likely to bare my teeth at you like a junkyard dog. Before dismissing me—or the dog—as ill-tempered, poorly trained, or not deserving of taking up space on this earth, stop for a moment and consider what might have happened in the prior ten or fifteen days, ten or fifteen weeks, or ten or fifteen years to prompt that reaction.

For at least an hour or two after a bad skate, I'm an open wound. Almost anything you say to me is going to hit me like salt. It's bad enough that I am required to engage with the media during this time. Anyone who insists on making contact can count on hearing something to the effect of: *I'm fucking really reactive right now and I have to skate in an exhibition with all the people who did really well. My less-than-stellar result has put me behind going into next season, and anything you have to say that doesn't recognize these realities is going to trigger my frustration, so please fuck off and leave me alone to process the fallout in peace and misery.*

I've always preferred to work through my demons on my own time, at my own pace, which explains a lot of the conflict between me and my mom, whose nurturing instinct was to try to "fix" things and make everything better. I realize there are better ways to handle disappointment, and I eventually do see the light and positivity in any situation, but only after beating myself up over my shortcomings. I just need to sit with my big feelings for an hour or two before I reengage with the world.

My friends know this about me. They are clear that I appreciate their kind words and outreach, but not immediately after a tragic performance, and they do their best to give me the space I need to have my little pity party. But sometimes they just can't help themselves. A dear friend who is a former skater texted me after my free skate and then made matters a hundred times worse by saying that my performance didn't change the fact that I'm extraordinarily talented.

"Talented" is a nails-on-the-chalkboard word for me. Telling me I'm talented is saying that I won the genetic lottery. Same thing with "pretty." I don't have control over the length of my torso or how my features are arranged on my face. I sometimes wish I were seen as less talented, because then I wouldn't feel like I've squandered this gift from God every time I come up short. Any success I achieved would be ascribed to how hard I work.

In the spirit of having no more fucks to give, I tapped out a sarcasm-laced reply: "I decided to give myself six months to fig-ure it out before I see if I want to kill myself or not." I followed it up with another sarcastic text about James: "I love him to pieces but if I'm going to stick around there's no reason to bring him down with me." And then I blocked her. The shame I feel when I beat up on those who only want to help me can turn my two-hour pity party into a weekend rager. I'm eventually open to peo-ple's feedback, but getting to that point is often exhausting. It takes a toll on everyone around me.

The first words I spoke to James in Nashville, long after we had arrived back at the hotel, was a request. Could we have McDon-ald's? The quality of food I was putting in my body didn't matter since I was absolutely, positively done skating.

Once upon a time I had been first in the country and fourth in the world. But now nine Americans were better than me. It was time to go home, drink peach whiskey in the dark (mango margs are reserved for happy occasions), and move on with my life. I wouldn't be in Beijing. But those Olympics would find me and drag me back into the past in the most excruciating way. They would call into question my most basic and abiding assumptions about the sport.

22

MAGIC PILLS

Everybody was mesmerized by Kamila Valieva's balletic lines and extension, her spins and combinations, and her quadruple Salchow in the short program, the first four-rotation jump landed by a woman at an Olympics.

From my vantage point—on the couch at my coach's house, seven thousand miles from the 2022 Winter Olympics in Beijing, China—I couldn't get past Kamila's cut, ripped arms and her veins, as visible as stocking seams. Skaters use their arms even less than soccer players. There's no reason for them to be so . . . *sinewy.* My eating disorder and body dysmorphia demons were jealous.

I wondered: How was it that all the Russian women singles skaters looked like dairy maids who churn butter and milk cows between ice sessions?

I couldn't unsee those arms.

Kamila propelled Russia to victory in the team event. What happened next is why nobody should look at the Russians and pretend that there's nothing to see there.

By the end of the Games, Kamila was engulfed in a doping scandal for having tested positive two months earlier for trimetazidine, the same banned substance that would subsequently be found in the urine of a Kenyan distance runner.

Think about it. Where does the Venn diagram of a skater and distance runner intersect? My best guess is in the stamina that a runner needs to avoid the proverbial wall late in a race and that a skater needs to cleanly land a quad or a triple Lutz–triple toe loop combination late in a free skate.

The doping revelation undammed a river of hypotheticals in my mind: What if the gold medalist in Sochi, Adelina Sotnikova, had been a pawn in Russia's doping system? Adelina roiled the waters when she acknowledged in a July 2023 interview on a YouTube channel that she failed a drug test at the Sochi Olympics. "I was supposed to have a trial, but I was acquitted because the second sample was opened and everything was fine," she said.

Yeah, no. Anybody who watched the 2017 documentary *Icarus* is aware that a system was in place in Sochi in which the Russians' dirty urine was subbed out for clean urine that had been collected before the competition. Adelina's explanation doesn't absolve her of guilt. To the contrary, it opens a Pandora's pee cup.

What if I was really the third-best skater in Sochi? What if the 2014 Olympics had been held in Salzburg, Austria, instead of Sochi? What if Evgenia Medvedeva and Anna Pogorilaya were not clean at the 2016 World Championships?

It's thought-provoking, but ultimately pointless, to ride the raging current of regret or outrage, to wonder how my late teens and twenties might have unfolded differently if I had won two medals in Sochi to join Beatrix Loughran, Tenley Albright, Carol Heiss Jenkins, Nancy Kerrigan, and Michelle Kwan as the only U.S. ladies' singles skaters to earn at least two career Olympic medals (Beatrix also won a medal in pairs).

I would have been in pretty exclusive company. Just saying.

That second medal would have changed my life. No doubt about it. What I'll never know is, would it have been for better or worse? I've made my peace with the situation. I look back at 2014 with genuine pride. I'm more than happy that I finished fourth in a field that included Yuna Kim, Mao Asada, Carolina Kostner, and so many other incredible athletes.

I'm a firm believer that life follows some cosmic design that is unknowable because each of us holds only one piece of the grand puzzle. But in the Olympic universe the people in charge certainly have enough bits of information to see that the competitive playing field is not level. The cheaters are winning, and I don't mean a rogue athlete here and there.

The Russians' systemic use of performance-enhancing drugs was first brought to light by German documentarians in December 2014, when Valieva would have been eight years old. As more details surfaced and Valieva's participation in the women's singles was up in the air, my mind traveled back to the doping control center in Sochi. I was escorted by a uniformed official with the World Anti-Doping Agency (WADA) to provide a urine sample. It's a routine procedure, but I remember this experience being strange. For example, doping control centers are usually like rooms at chain hotels. They look the same no matter where in the world you are. The one in Sochi stood out in my memory because from the moment I stepped inside, it had a different vibe. I distinctly recall thinking, *This looks more like an informal cocktail reception than doping control.*

An unusual number of people were milling around who were not wearing shirts and jackets with the official WADA logo. There were more men than I'm accustomed to seeing in what is supposed to be a very private, very regimented space. It never crossed my mind that anything shady could be going on. For someone who grew up in a family where shady things were happening under my nose, I remain surprisingly trusting. Or maybe just naive. You don't see what you're not looking for, and since it never occurred to me to cheat, I didn't picture anyone else doing it.

Nobody with any power in sport seems inclined to mess with Russia, which enjoys an outsized influence in figure skating administration, is the biggest exporter of coaches, and at the Olympics since 1964 has won 53 percent of all the medals (forty-one of seventy-eight) in ice dancing and pairs skating.

And over the past decade, its dominance has spilled into my event. After Adelina became the first Russian to win the women's singles, Russian-born women have won both the subsequent Olympic singles' titles. The coach credited with opening the floodgates is a retired ice dancer named Eteri Tutberidze, whose methods are questionable at best but who has such powerful allies I reflexively glanced over my shoulder before typing her name.

Eteri's athletes have been rumored to train over ten hours a day, six days a week. That's what filtered back to us in the United States, which has the effect, intended or not, of making us question whether we're too soft physically or mentally or both to compete with the Russians.

Eteri—who generally denies any wrongdoing—was open about her athletes' use of meldonium, which she described as a "recovery drug" (it has since been banned by the World Anti-Doping Agency). Have I mentioned my recovery drug? It's called sleep, and I definitely could stand to increase my dosage.

For the record, those training stories never passed my smell test. From experience, I know how my skating deteriorates in the third hour of an on-ice session. The idea that anyone could last more than twice that amount of time was inconceivable to me. It made me envious. I remember joking that I wished there was a magic pill that would allow me to train for that long and recover quickly enough that I could do it all over again the next day.

I had no idea that that joke was nibbling around the edges of the truth. The revelation of a state-sponsored doping system helped it all make sense to me, though in fairness, none of the first two dozen Russians banned for doping offenses in the wake of the 2014 Sochi scandal were figure skaters. The Russians had discovered a really effective shortcut, and while all the women I've competed against, including Adelina, steadfastly deny any wrongdoing, my bullshit detector is on high alert. Especially Kamila, a child, tested positive for a heart drug prescribed for angina but used by athletes to improve blood flow and endurance—and was allowed to compete anyway.

Let me also say this. It's beyond ironic that I spent several years attempting to compete with the Russians' strength and stamina with starvation and laxatives. That's a headshaker.

Performance-enhancing drugs aren't something you take the day of an event, like sugar cubes back in the day, to give you a quick burst of energy. They're far more sophisticated and geared not for competition but for training, which is where the real magic happens.

See, the human body was not designed to go and go and go like an Energizer bunny. The longer a skater is able to train, the more their moves become second nature, and the more their moves become second nature, the more confidence they gain. Something I live-tweeted during the women's singles competition at the 2018 Olympics, which was dominated by Eteri's skaters, stands out in retrospect. Fifteen-year-old Alina Zagitova won the gold and eighteen-year-old Evgenia Medvedeva took the silver. Of Evgenia, I tweeted, "I can feel her confidence through my laptop."

Maybe this is a hot take, but at this point I'd be okay with letting the Russians continue their doping regimen, provided we could have access to the same stuff (assuming that the drugs are thoroughly vetted and can be determined not to have unintended long-term consequences).

Fuck it. I can do a quad in a harness fueled by copious amounts of caffeine. Let's see how high I could jump and how good I'd feel in the fourth minute of my free skate with a chemist's little helper. I'm joking–not joking.

I'm tired of being demure while the sport burns. My boyfriend is a big golf fan, and one of the players he likes is Rory McIlroy, from Northern Ireland. And he's not alone. Someone from my former management agency who saw her job as making me as nonthreatening and palatable to as wide a swath of the American public as possible praised McIlroy on Twitter for his impassioned, principled stand against the hypocrisies and controversies embroiling men's professional golf. This is the same person who plays a substantive role in sanitizing skaters' voices and stories in the name of marketability.

You can't have it both ways. Oh, wait. In the world of Olympic sports, that's not true. You actually can. How else to explain the International Olympic Committee's decision to ban Russia and its national flag from the 2018 and 2022 Winter Olympics but allow Russian athletes to participate as unaffiliated competitors in Pyeongchang and under the Russian Olympic Committee flag in Beijing?

I'm sorry, but I missed the penalty part of these measures. If Minnie Mouse were to compete under the Olympic flag, it wouldn't matter. Everyone would still associate her with Disney.

I don't blame Adelina and the other Russians. In my mind, they're as much victims of their system as their non-Russian competitors are. Sotnikova was seventeen years old in Sochi. Valieva was fifteen in Beijing. They had no agency over their skating careers. They followed the instructions of their coaches and doctors and administrators. If they were led astray to improve their performance, the spotlight should be on those adults who are controlling the kids like puppeteers.

I can't hate the Russians. They're following instructions from the adults they trust. They're like us in many respects. I remember competing in an event in Tokyo as a teenager, and afterward I found myself at a karaoke bar with a group of skaters that included the Russian Elizaveta Tuktamysheva, who was so much fun to be around. We were seated in a VIP section and, led by Elizaveta, drinking gin. It tasted horrible.

"How can you drink this stuff?" I asked her.

"Tastes like perfume," she agreed, smiling.

At some point, somebody at the table got the wild idea to do a topless toast while raising shot glasses, which precipitated us being shown the exit by bouncers.

Elizaveta was known as "The Empress." She would win a European championship and a world championship—and pose for a Russian men's magazine. But she never made an Olympic team, and she acknowledged taking meldonium before it was banned by WADA. The sanctity of sport rests on being able to trust that the results are legitimate. On knowing that the competitive playing field is level. In the Olympic realm, we've all but lost that. It sickened me to see Valieva's fourth-place finish in the women's event in Beijing being mined for ratings and internet clicks. It saddened me to see the silver medalist Alexandra Trusova, also from Russia, in hysterics backstage, screaming something to the effect of "Everyone has a gold medal. Everyone but me. I hate skating. I hate it."

A part of me wanted to beam myself through the screen and provide a human shield for Trusova from the camera's prying lens. Another part of me wanted to say to her, *How do you think the rest of us feel?*

We've had proof for nearly a decade that the country churning out champions has not been operating aboveboard. Russia has turned cheating into a high-level, intricate, almost art-form-level endeavor. The Russians have shown themselves to be the runaway gold medalists of doping. Congratulations to them! It's worth noting that since Russia's invasion of Ukraine in 2022, its skaters have been barred from international events. Not coincidentally, as they've been absent from competition, so too, for the most part have women's quad jumps.

I am so, so tired of being asked why the United States hasn't won a gold medal in women's singles since Sarah Hughes in 2002 or a medal of any color since Sasha Cohen in 2006. As time goes on, the U.S. women's medal drought no longer appears to be a blip, an oddity, an aberration. It's looking more and more like an expression of a climate change in the sport that threatens the Olympic dreams of young female American skaters and perhaps of clean skaters everywhere.

Instead of asking why the United States isn't getting better results, I'd argue that the better question is this: Should we aspire for our young skaters to be competitive with the Russians now that we know what it requires? And for what? A few headlines and a leading role in an ice show? It's certainly not for the money, because the financial returns on the sport, at least in America, are almost nil.

Observing the drama caused by skating's politics and the sport's corruption was helpful in reframing how I pictured my career. I realized that it would be silly to live out my days haunted by what might have been in Sochi. As a participant, I had viewed the Olympics as the pinnacle of sport. As a spectator, they came across more like a slickly produced reality TV show.

The 2022 Olympics also reinforced how much is out of the control of even the best skaters on the planet. I recognized the value of following a figure skater's serenity prayer. Why stress out about whether my scores would be fair, or whether my competitors were clean when I had only a limited ability to change the outcome? That context freed me of so much baggage that had been weighing me down, and it absolutely informed my decision to keep skating.

There were things I could change—and would in the coming months. Mainly, this time I would do it for myself, on my own terms, in the body that I, at long last, truly felt comfortable in.

23

GOT TO GET IT OFF MY CHEST

In the first years of my comeback, I had to add an extra step to my pre-competition routine—always in the privacy of my hotel room, so paranoid was I that my secret might be exposed. Before I slipped into my skating costume, applied my makeup, or swept my hair into a tight bun, I thoroughly taped my tits. If you look closely at the footage of my free skate at the 2020 or 2022 U.S. Championships, through the flesh-colored material in my costumes you can see the flesh-colored tape clearly visible above the rib cage. No one ever inquired about it, probably because nobody in the world of women's skating is going to look at KT Tape and think, *Oooh, a DIY chest binding!*

The taping process tacked on another thirty minutes to an hour of prep time, but I didn't have a choice. As much as I sweated my opening triple-triple combination or double Axel, my biggest source of anxiety was my chest binding. Did I apply enough tape? Did it look normal? Would my tits remain secured while I was skating? Would I be able to breathe well enough to complete my long program?

More than a fall, I dreaded sinking into a sit spin only to have one of my girls, yearning to be free, wiggle loose and oscillate half a revolution behind my body. These were new worries because the body I inhabited starting around 2017 was significantly curvier than in the days when I was starving myself.

My flat chest had enabled my jumps because I was more streamlined in the air. This advantage never crossed my mind until I began packing on the pounds in Detroit, became top-heavy, and my center of gravity changed. Waking up one day with two triple-Ds was wild. That's not exactly how it happened. It just felt that way.

Wilder still, I noticed that men started appraising me differently. Women, too. It was discomfiting to not want this Jessica Rabbit figure that so many men clearly found desirable and so many women let me know they envied. I had no illusions. In the skating world, I knew that my tits, if anybody got a peek at them, would be viewed as a vulgar symbol of my inability to conquer my appetite and exert control over my body.

Can we be honest? Spot reduction is a myth. As I lost weight post-recovery, it became painfully obvious that there was no fitness or diet strategy to help me lose the pounds in my chest, which I identified as my most troublesome area. I lost more than fifty pounds, none of it from my chest, and gained the clarity that I was never going to return to a B cup.

Sports bras didn't work for me, because most of them are made of stretchy material and are designed to support or lift the girls up, not to strap them down. My goal was to suffocate my chest, not give the girls room to breathe. While scouring online sites for options, I fell down a rabbit hole that led me to tape used by transgender individuals. Of course! It made total sense. Who else would be similarly invested in making their chests as small as possible and eliminating all cleavage?

I studied online tutorials on how to use the rolls of kinesiology tape, made from materials advertised as soft and breathable. Breathable? Not so much. But what was a big-chested gal in a flat-chested sport going to do? I devoured all the helpful tips. I made sure my chest was dry before I applied the tape and waited to use deodorant until afterward so the taping would stick. I added a small bottle of baby oil to my toiletries kit in case I had trouble removing the tape once I was back in the hotel after a competition. Along the way, I gained a deep appreciation for the painstaking and painful steps that some female-to-male members of the trans community endure every day to be able to move through the world more comfortably.

I had to laugh when one of the videos, as part of its promotional pitch, said, "So you can dance the night away without worrying about a wardrobe malfunction." I just wanted to be able to skate four minutes without a nip slip. Or without the girls bouncing around during my jumps. You can cross your arms over your chest before you run down a flight of stairs, but not as you step into a triple Lutz.

To be on the safe side, I'd sometimes stick with chest binders, which are like a compression sleeve for your boobs. The packaging label explicitly states not to exercise while wearing one because it restricts breathing and advises against wearing one for more than six hours at a time. I read a lot of literature that presented chest binders as dangerous and medically unsafe. I ignored it.

I had no choice. For me, having my chest strapped so that I could perform better superseded any comfort issues. My breathing did become more shallow, but it wasn't anything I couldn't endure. And I got used to it after a while. Carly tried on one of my chest binders before a hockey game and didn't even make it onto the ice before discarding it. "How do you wear this?" she gasped.

It's a bitch, I agreed. Not fun. But functionally necessary. Having a huge chest in a sport where I was surrounded by pre-pubescent bodies impacted me in other ways. Because I was self-conscious about my curves, my posture suffered because I slouched, folding into myself. I expended so much mental energy and put so much fucking work into managing something for which there was a medical solution.

My mother had chest reduction surgery back when the procedure was more archaic. Modern medicine's advances have made the operation much less of a butchery. Because my mother's default mindset is worst-case scenarios, I didn't share my plans with her. I chose to operate under the assumption that it's better to ask for forgiveness than permission.

I wanted the surgery despite our culture's obsession with big boobs. I wanted the surgery even though I knew there would be people who would equate my feelings about my large chest with my complicated relationship with my weight and body image. A psychologist cut right to the heart of the matter, as she saw it: Did I view the procedure as a way to lose another six or seven pesky pounds?

It was wearisome having to justify why I was desperate to have this surgery. If you have a nose job because you are having trouble breathing, it's not considered cosmetic. But if you have a boob job because you are experiencing excruciating back and shoulder pain, that's elective?

The distinction, of course, is that we live in a world where women's breasts are sexualized and objectified, making it hard to talk about them in unemotional terms. In a culture that equates breast size with beauty and prizes men's desires above everything else, having reduction surgery is seen as frivolous. Or, worse, as a modern-day form of self-mutilation. It's still hard in a world that is supposedly all about body positivity to say, *Hey, I have this de-*

sirable feature, but it's ruining my life and causing me daily pain. People react as if it is—or I am—a punch line.

My hope in bringing it up here is that the next person who finds themselves in my position will be shown more compassion. That they won't be completely misunderstood by roughly 80 percent of women and 100 percent of men.

Chest size and its impact on exercise is absolutely a conversation worth starting. Research has shown that discomfort from the size of one's chest or bra fit can be a deterrent to exercising. I stumbled upon a 2019 study published in the *Journal of Science and Medicine in Sport* that found that as women's breast sizes grew, their participation in physical exercise, especially if it was strenuous, decreased. In James's homeland, the United Kingdom, a 2016 study of over two thousand girls ages eleven through seventeen found that 73 percent reported having at least one breast-related concern as it relates to sport and exercise.

I debated whether to have the surgery for far too long because of the stigma. I remember floating the idea a few times in what I believed to be friendly company only to be told that I must be "crazy" or "ungrateful." More than one person said something to the effect of, "Most people pay for big tits like yours and you want to cut them off? You can't. That's ridiculous."

Forget our uteruses. It's as if the concept "my body, my choice" doesn't exist when it comes to our chests.

After the 2022 nationals, my path became clear. I was determined to have the surgery one way or the other. My decision was based solely on health concerns. I needed to give my back and shoulders a break. The performance piece didn't enter the equation since I had no plan to continue skating.

The cost was my main concern. I wasn't sure I could come up with enough money for the procedure, even though I didn't think I could afford *not* to have it done. I considered selling the exclu-

sive rights to the story of my reduction surgery to a weekly tabloid to finance it. I was determined to do whatever it took. I
talked it over with my agent, Tara, and it turns out she grew up
with a plastic surgeon based on Long Island. She made a call to
him on my behalf. It was kismet. He came highly recommended,
he was affordable, and, miraculously, he had an opening in
March.

I rode the train from Philadelphia to New York for an evaluation with the surgeon. After the examination, he leveled with me.
He had watched me perform at nationals, and based on that eyeball assessment he'd been prepared to try to talk me out of the
surgery. But he did a complete 180 after examining my narrow
rib cage and my "Snoopy-nose-shaped" breasts resting low on
my frame, as if they had been drawn onto my body by the car-
toonist Charles Schulz.

The surgery was relatively straightforward. I had an anesthesiologist who was delightful. She was also a woman, so I didn't
have to risk the potentially nightmarish scenario of imagining
my dad's face smothering mine with gas.

I woke up in the recovery room feeling sick to my stomach. I
am not good with anesthesia. I knew from my post-surgery experience having my wisdom teeth pulled years prior that I had
about thirty minutes tops before I was going to hurl my brains
out. Tara was the first person I saw when I woke up, and I told her
that I was dizzy and that if she didn't get me to the hotel where I
was spending the night, and fast, I probably was going to puke in
her car.

I made it to the hotel room before I threw up. I was pretty out
of it for a few days. I had a ten-day Percocet prescription for the
pain, but I stopped two days in after scaring James to death when
I woke up in the middle of the night sobbing because I was so
dizzy.

I didn't expect to have any regrets about the surgery. I had done my research, read dozens of first-person accounts, and not a single one described the procedure as anything but the best decision they ever made. I'm eternally grateful to Tara for helping make the surgery happen. And to James for encouraging me to go ahead with the procedure when I was entertaining second and third thoughts because of the cost. Both assured me that it would pay off every single day in terms of my basic comfort.

And if I didn't have the surgery now, when?

As the bruises faded, a clear picture emerged of what my life would look like moving forward. Every top I tried on fit infinitely better; they didn't dig into the flesh below my armpits.

In the spring, I headlined an ice show. I had my costume fittings two months after the surgery, and something that used to be a royal pain was pure joy. Being able to change backstage between numbers was also so much easier. No taping, no hassle. No more performing in something so tight I couldn't breathe. I simply put on a regular sports bra like other women and did my number like everybody else.

It was freeing. James was in the audience for a couple of my shows. Many days he was on the ice at the same time as me. From either vantage point, what stood out the most to him was how comfortable I looked. My spins were a little faster. My revolutions were tighter. He was the first one to say out loud what I had been thinking: "You should skate one more season," he said. "You should try competing again in this body that you feel so much more comfortable in."

I did feel lighter, but I can't attribute it solely to the surgery. My chest wasn't the only things weighing me down that I decided to address.

24

GROWN-UP GOLD

Our family portraits remind me of the inkblots in the famous Rorschach test. From birth until I was twenty-one, I saw my parents one way, and I wouldn't have believed it possible to perceive them any differently. Then their behavior became more erratic, and I realized that the conservative, strict, rule-following Christian household I grew up in was a facade. That realization changed how I looked at them. How I looked at everything.

The work that I began in treatment and which is ongoing is all about processing my mom and dad through an adult's eyes instead of through my child and adolescent brain. To blame myself for my parents' marital discord, as I did for so long, was misguided. I can see that now.

My job moving forward is not to idealize my mom, dad, and sister or try to change them or wish they had been different. To heal myself, I have to look at them honestly, accept them unconditionally, and determine what a healthy relationship with them should look like. It has been a hard, and sometimes painful, process of discovery.

Skating for me is the way and the truth and the life, and it felt particularly *holy* on one of those crisp winter days in Manhattan that make the Big Apple so delectable. It was December 2019, and I was circling the ice like a sugarplum fairy on a temporary rink at Bryant Park. I was there on behalf of one of my sponsors, smiling and styling and spinning and grinning and feeling in general like all was right with the world, when a voice commanded my attention: "Gracie! Gracie!"

I skated another lap. "Gracie! Gracie!" I turned my head in the direction of the voice and did a double take. My mind was buzzing with questions. How did he know where I was? Why had he come? And who was the woman he was standing next to all cozy-like?

My agent observed me skate over and speak to the man who seconds earlier had been shouting my name like some deranged fan, and she noted the fake smile frozen on my face. Her mama bear instincts kicked into high gear and she hurried over to rescue me. You can imagine her surprise when I said, "Tara, meet my dad." She audibly gasped.

Dad appeared genuinely perplexed that I wasn't delighted to see him. He never was adept at picking up even the most obvious social cues. I had been ignoring most of his texts and voice messages since our previous encounter, a stilted dinner around the time of the 2018 Olympics. I don't know why he thought showing up unannounced to see me was the right play.

I agreed to have dinner with him that night but brought two friends for moral support. The three of us listened in bored silence as Dad talked about his jobs selling medical equipment and moonlighting as an Uber driver. He was stricken when I didn't praise him for getting a new job after stealing urine, suing the

Illinois Board of Medicine, and going several months without telling his family that he had been suspended. At one point I remember him saying I should be proud of him for "getting back out there" and "not staying in bed all day being depressed." Was that a shot at me and my black hole of an existence in Detroit? One of my friends thought so. When the three of us were safely back in the car, she said, "I see what you mean. Your father really does have an ability to make you feel like shit."

There was a time I would have agreed with her. But by 2019 I recognized that he couldn't make me feel shitty without my permission—and I wasn't granting it. There's no Hallmark greeting card to express the complicated feelings I have for him. The front would have to read "Fuck. Off." And inside: "I do not forgive you."

My dad has never apologized for losing his job because of his prescription pill addiction, has never accepted responsibility for his actions or sought to make reparations to the people he hurt. Part of me thinks he could bridge the gulf between us with a simple "I'm sorry," but another part of me believes that he still doesn't think he did anything wrong. He continues to view himself as the victim.

Given what I've been through, I'm the last person to judge anybody's worst impulses. I appreciate that in Dad's chosen field, anesthesiology, the potential for abusing the drugs you administer is real. So much so that it's a topic that would have been broached during his training. For those whose job it is to deliver people to a state of peacefulness not easily reached in the conscious world, turning such awesome powers on yourself must be really seductive.

But my dad's inability to acknowledge that he messed up and his refusal to say that he's sorry tell me everything I need to know. Why am I expected to forgive him without any change on his part? Why am I the one who is supposed to apologize for not maintaining our relationship? It's so messed up. In 2022, I neglected to wish him a happy Father's Day, and he responded with a text-based charm offensive:

"Hi, hoping you are okay. Haven't heard from you in a while. I think about you every day and love you so much. Oh, well, you are my daughter. I love you. It's more important to be close when times are not so good." He included a photo of us from when I was a child. He mentioned he was going to be in Philadelphia on business and would love to stay with me. Never mind that my apartment has one bedroom. Unless he expected to sleep in the bathtub, I don't know what he was thinking.

Every three days, like clockwork, he texted me, asking for a chance to talk and saying he really needed family. I still didn't reply, so he sent the same text string again. And again. And again. He called and left a voicemail saying that many therapists would recommend that we see each other.

Yeah, no. Any half-decent therapist would not recommend continuing to make contact with someone who clearly doesn't wish to engage. There's a word for that kind of behavior: "harassment."

Dad wasn't done: "Last chance to respond, pretty please. Last, last chance."

And then, finally: "I don't know why you're icing me."

So very many words, and not one sentence inquiring about my well-being. It was all about him. It always has been. Sometimes I'd read his maudlin texts about how alone he is and how much I mean to him and I'd feel bad. But I couldn't shake the suspicion that Dad doesn't actually love or miss me. He loves and misses the extension of himself that is the skater Gracie Gold, and he's trying to manipulate me to be a part of his life again. Because what's more validating to his ego than seeing himself reflected in his famous and special daughter?

As my father drama was playing out in one room, James sat slumped in the other room, struggling to come to grips with the fact that back in Britain, the father he adored was fading fast. It was an uncomfortable irony lost on neither of us that I was blowing off my dad, who is very much alive, while James was desperate to make contact with his dad, who would soon be dead.

I did my best to walk with James in his grief. I knew better than to confuse his pain for the father he lost with my pain for the father I lack. James and I talked about it. He asked me, "What if you're estranged from your dad when he dies? How will you feel?" James made it home to London and was holding his father's hand when he drew his last breath. It was a profound experience for him, so my apathy toward my dad is hard for him to comprehend.

"I'd be sad, too, to lose a dad if I had one like yours," I said. "But you can't think of my dad and picture yours, because we grew up with totally different fathers." In any case, my conscience is clear. When I contemplate my relationship with my dad, the truest sentiments I can muster are ones I'd have to borrow from a Noah Kahan song: "So I thought that if I piled something good on all my bad / That I could cancel out the darkness I inherited from Dad."

Carly couldn't get off work to attend Skate America in 2022, so I had Mom all to myself in Boston. It was a pleasant experience, actually. We met for coffee, and then James joined us for dinner and ably filled the tension-defusing role normally played by Carly. Skating events are a minefield for me and Mom. They amplify the distance between us. Mom clearly wants to be part of my journey and lighten my load, but she doesn't want to overstep. And I want her to be part of my journey, too, but have a hard time establishing healthy boundaries.

We're both so afraid of saying the wrong thing that our conversations never get past the surface. We talk a lot about our art projects. At times it feels like we are miles apart. But there are signs that the gap is closing.

Mom returned to work after I left for Detroit in 2017. She was in her sixties, an age when most of her friends were retiring and becoming snowbirds or golfers or cruise-goers. She had no choice. Dad had lost his hospital job, temporarily at first and then permanently, and my skating at that point certainly wasn't bringing in much ancillary income.

She was still settling in on the overnight shift at a hospital in Long Beach, California, when I called her. We hadn't been on the phone long, maybe five minutes, when she confessed that I had caught her at a bad time and that she really should hang up because she was up to her ears in paperwork.

"What kind of paperwork?" I asked.

"Oh, I got kicked in the face by a patient," she said, "so there are all these forms I have to fill out."

Wait. What? "I'm sorry, Mom," I said, "but you didn't think maybe to lead with that little piece of information?"

That's so on-brand for her—to casually slip into a conversation, almost as an aside, that she was attacked by a patient in the psych ward. She could make light of the incident, but it deeply bothered me that Mom had to spend her retirement years working. I felt like I had put her in the path of that violent patient, however indirectly. If I had been able to keep my shit together through the 2018 Olympics, I probably would have been able to support us.

But there was a silver lining to Mom's work. It gave her days structure, which she lacked in 2016 when her nest was emptying and she didn't know what to do with herself. Until then, Mom's every waking hour had revolved around us. She had thrown herself into parenting with the zeal of a recovering latchkey kid.

I have been critical of my mom for some of her decisions and actions. But what I've learned over the past few years has helped me see her in a much more sympathetic light. When I consider my mom's plight in late 1994—processing my dad's fentanyl addiction while newly pregnant with twins that they went to great lengths to conceive—my heart aches for her. It was a messed-up situation. I can see clearly now that their marriage was the biggest of Mom's reclamation projects, and she did her best to salvage it and turn it into something attractive.

And the bottom line is, with precious little help from her husband, Mom raised two very successful children. Would I be a two-time national champion and Olympic medalist if she didn't push us as hard as she did? Would Carly be a college graduate and financial adviser without Mom's prodding? It's hard to say, but if I had to hazard a guess, I'd say probably not.

Without Denise Gold, there is no Gracie Gold. The person or the performer. And Mom gave me Carly, who, with apologies to James, is my favorite person in the whole wide world. As long as I have Carly, I'll want for nothing.

As we've moved further into our twenties, Carly and I have grown more independent. We're less involved in each other's day-to-day lives, which makes the time we do spend together extra special. As our twenty-seventh birthdays approached in 2022, Carly suggested that we celebrate together in Southern California. She's the family social director, so I didn't think much of the fact that she took the lead on the planning and was weirdly persistent about making sure I locked in my travel arrangements. But then I earned an invitation to Champs Camp, which was taking place around the same time as our birthdays and I had to cancel. I was disappointed, but Carly was nearly inconsolable. How weird, I thought. I rebooked my trip to California for the Christmas holiday. Carly could hardly wait to give me her present.

I tore open the box, pulled aside the tissue, and couldn't believe my eyes. Carly had hunted for a replacement for Blankie upon noticing that he was looking a little worse for the wear after more than a quarter of a century of faithful service. After scouring online sites for months, she had struck pay dirt on eBay.

I was overjoyed. It was such a thoughtful gift, the best present ever. Carly explained that the blanket was supposed to be for my birthday, which was why she'd been so crestfallen when I couldn't come to California to celebrate it. She wanted to see my face when I opened it, so she set it aside until my next visit.

We immediately made plans to mark our twenty-eighth birthdays with matching tattoos of the blanket's balloon-wielding bunny. We are so in sync, almost telepathically so, that I can't say that I was surprised when I called Carly to tell her I had broken my left foot and she informed me that she had broken her collarbone playing in her adult hockey rec league.

It's been a long time since Carly had to put up with fans who pulled their faces into expressions of sympathy when they saw us together, stared at Carly, and said, "It must be so hard to be her sister."

She thought it was hilarious. I was less amused. I'd smile, but inside I was cringing. I remember thinking every single time it happened, *What the fuck? Am I that big of a monster?*

What's really funny is that Carly is enjoying the last laugh. She's the one who retired from skating on her own terms. She's the one who enrolled in college and got busy on her next act. It has become crystal clear to me, if not to our parents or skating fans, that I'm not the tough act to follow. Carly is. And every year I feel as if I keep losing ground to her.

As an adult, I've established healthier boundaries with all of my family members to maintain my emotional health and well-being. Skating competitively on my own, without my parents' financial backing or emotional investment, has been instructive. Being able to perform for my own reasons, with no one else's gratification tied up in the results, has thrown into sharp relief all the ways that skating infected our family.

It was like a virus that fed on insecurities created by the sport's sheer expense and demands for perfectionism. From almost the beginning, the message underscoring every move was that the Olympics and lucrative ice shows are the endgame and if I wasn't chasing those, what was the point of skating? Of existing?

Now that I'm skating for myself, I can see clearly how tangled the family ties can become when extrinsic rewards—medals and pro contracts, for example—become the goal. There's nothing inherently wrong with having lofty ambitions if the sport is kept in the proper perspective, which isn't easy to do.

If sports federations and families learn nothing else from my story, I hope it's that steeping children in a competitive cauldron that prioritizes prizes and riches over their well-being is a prescription for sadness—and for trouble.

25

"I'LL BE BACK"

My showing at the 2022 nationals left me in limbo. Tenth place wasn't the mic-drop I had hoped for in my comeback, so what did I have to gain by continuing? I embarked on my Ice Dreams tour with no expectations or agenda other than to enjoy each performance.

My chest reduction surgery gave me the motivation to keep going, but I didn't want to commit to anything. During our downtime between shows, my friend Michael Solonoski helped me choreograph a new long program just in case. I was hedging my bets. Less than three weeks after we pieced it together, I impulsively decided to officially unveil it at the Philadelphia Summer Invitational, a minor event with a strong field at my home rink, IceWorks.

To my surprised delight, I landed five triples, including the triple Lutz–triple toe combination, in my free skate on the way to a third-place overall finish. It was my first podium appearance in *forever*. Put it this way: The last time it had happened, President Obama occupied the White House.

As I stood with the bronze medal around my neck, my smile was incandescent. Michael said he had never seen me so happy. He whipped out his phone and snapped a photograph to commemorate the occasion. He showed me the image, and I had to admit it: Joy becomes me.

The photo jarred loose a memory from the 2014 Olympics. I'd told Frank that I wanted to throw my team Olympic bronze medal into the trash because it wasn't a gold. Can you imagine? What was *wrong* with me? I mean, tell me you're a pathological perfectionist without telling me you're a pathological perfectionist.

With my podium showing, I earned an invitation to Champs Camp. It was a big deal. Just when I figured I'd be walking away from the sport, I had worked my way back into America's elite skating mix. If 1 million people had returned to skating from my 2017 rock bottom, 999,999 probably wouldn't have lasted more than a few weeks. A few months, tops. I wore my perseverance like a badge of honor. It was all good, except that Champs Camp was being held in . . . Detroit. (If this had been a movie, I would have arched my eyebrows and said, "A little too on-the-nose.") But ready or not, I booked my return to my Waterloo.

At least we trained at Detroit Skating Club, which was nowhere near my old neighborhood. The arena triggered no terrible memories. If I could take the emotion out of it, Detroit was preferable to Colorado Springs. I was spared the altitude and the army-barracks-style dorms, both of which could be real downers. I checked into a comfortable hotel and approached the weekend with the attitude that it could go either way. I could be very good or horrid. The beauty for me was that I would have been at peace with either outcome.

I wouldn't say that I nailed both my programs, but one judge said I came across as "grounded and grateful," and the technical expert declared my jumps "clean," which made my heart soar. At the end of camp, I won a skate-off to secure two international assignments: Nebelhorn Trophy and Skate America. Seven months after I was presumed done, I had new life.

My skating between June and August was intense. It was the best I'd trained in years. It felt as if my coaches and I had figured out the recipe, the perfect mix between pushing my body and preserving it. All my hard work was coming together in a rewarding-as-fuck fashion. Then, during a routine practice in the summer of 2022, I fell several times, as one does, and woke up the next day with full-out pain in my glute. My right hip throbbed. Injuries are an occupational hazard for every athlete, but this was a setback I could ill afford. I didn't have time to heal. It was particularly frustrating to have my mind and body out of sync—again. What a cruel joke to have spent my teens in great physical shape but with a rickety psyche, only to shore up my mental deficiencies and have my body fail me.

I was twelfth in the fifteen-woman field at the Nebelhorn Trophy. From the moment I stepped foot in Oberstdorf, Germany, I felt off. I hadn't arranged my travel to allow my body to acclimate to the time change, and though the judges responded positively to my skating in practices, I couldn't shake my sluggishness on the ice—or my hip pain. In the short program, I fell on my money jump, the triple Lutz, which was mortifying. The competition went downhill from there.

I had no time to feel sorry for myself because Skate America was right around the corner. I had much to prove in Boston: that I could move past that dismal performance in Germany; that I would not be haunted by my last event in Boston, that fourth-place finish at the 2016 worlds; that I could rise above my injury.

For all intents and purposes, Skate America was my first international Grand Prix assignment since the 2018 Rostelecom Cup

in Russia, where I pulled out after the short program. I'd participated in Skate America in 2020, but it was limited to U.S. competitors because of COVID-19 restrictions. The 2022 edition
featured a formidable international field that included the reigning world champion and 2022 Olympic bronze medalist, Kaori
Sakamoto of Japan, whose skating I had admired from afar.

The event was held at an arena in the Boston suburb of Nor-
wood. Thank goodness for small favors. At least I didn't have to
negotiate the TD Garden ice again. I was the oldest competitor in
women's singles, which meant that I brought a wealth of experience to the ice. On the flip side, it meant my muscle memory
contained layers of scar tissue.

My practice sessions produced endless chatter, most of it positive. People remarked on how relaxed and confident I looked. I
was consistently landing my triples. It was a sign of how good
I felt that before I stepped on the ice for my short program, I
slipped off my gloves, which are not just decorative. They make
me feel more like I do in practice, and for some reason during the
last year or two I'd hated taking them off. (One of my weird sensory issues, perhaps?) By removing them I was telling everybody,
I've got this.

I skated a nearly perfect program. I was the only woman in the
field to pull off a flawless triple Lutz–triple toe combination. The.
Only. One. I felt more in command of that combination than I
had in Sochi. In my performances, my expressions are another
part of the choreography; I smile here, I make eye contact with
the judging panel there. This was one of the rare times when my
smile was organic, a natural byproduct of the joy I felt because I
was connecting to the ice *and* the music *and* the audience. That
smile could not be knocked from my face even when, in my excitement, I took off too quickly on a triple loop late in the program and fell. It was the only nit I could pick with the program.

With a fifth-place finish, I secured a spot in the final group of skaters for the long program.

I long ago abandoned social media because my body dysmorphia almost guarantees that I will be distressed by the photographs posted of me. And life is too short to waste one second of it reading hateful comments by strangers like "Hi, Flabby." I mostly leave it to my agent and my boyfriend to monitor my social media accounts. After the short program they reported back that the reaction of the public was overwhelmingly positive. The praise came fast and furious. I was described as a great technician. As the best technician that the U.S. women have ever produced. I was described as a "legend." Praised for my grace. People spoke of "cheer crying" as they watched me.

It was gratifying. I was *pumped.* To have gone out and performed better than most people probably believed was possible at my age—reports after the fact made it seem like, at twenty-seven, I'd risen from my deathbed to deliver the performance—was exhilarating. I was reminded why I love skating so much.

The skating culture is another story. When I met with reporters after my beautiful, evocative, technically sound program, one of the first questions I fielded was about my physical appearance.

"You look like you're in really good shape," said the reporter who then asked about my conditioning regimen.

I don't know why, after so many years negotiating so many mixed zones, I was surprised, but it took all of my training to keep my smile, now frozen stiff, affixed to my face.

When will people in skating realize that affirmative comments about a skater's looks are not the antidote to disordered eating but actually can help perpetuate it? Any—I repeat, *any*—comments about physical appearance can reinforce body dysmorphia. Please, please, *please,* I know you believe you are paying me a compliment, but can we keep the focus on the quality of my jumps or the personal significance of my Grand Prix return?

It was discouraging to note that when it came to my body, it was still form over function.

My free skate the next day was far from perfect—no surprise given that my glute injury had severely limited how much I had been able to train since returning from Detroit. I was sucking wind pretty badly by the fourth minute. I ended up sixth overall, four places behind Isabeau Levito, who was second in her Grand Prix debut. Kaori Sakamoto, at twenty-two a grown-up like me, was crowned the champion. *Adults skate, too!*

I had little time to regroup before I headed to Graz, Austria, for a third international assignment. Graz is a picturesque place that's renowned for its art, design, and architecture. But that's not why I was thrilled to be going there, even if a transatlantic flight was the last thing the orthopedist would have recommended for my deteriorating right hip. (Next to competing, that is, since at this point I could hardly rotate to the right with my torso—the treatment wasn't working—and I'd become someone in chronic pain with no relief in sight.)

It was my first trip back to Graz since Polina Edmunds, Ashley Wagner, and I had been sequestered there for ten days between the team event and the ladies' singles at the 2014 Olympics. Eight years later, Polina and Ashley were long since retired, and I had no business, really, returning to the city whose attractions include a museum devoted to local son Arnold Schwarzenegger. And yet there I was.

How many times since I emerged from recovery had I parroted Schwarzenegger's signature line from *The Terminator*, "I'll be back"? But I never could have imagined returning *here*, where I'd spent a sliver of my most celebrated winter. It took a summer in which I delivered my most inspired skating in several years to earn this fall Challenger Series assignment. It was another big step in my journey to reclaim my past.

The symbolism wasn't lost on me as I started out from the hotel where Polina, Ashley, and I had stayed in 2014. Using a photograph from that time to orient myself, I retraced our steps to the side of the bridge over the River Mur, where I thought I might find the lock that we had left, provided it had not succumbed to the elements. (I did note that the Hooters where I had eaten every meal had closed down, a casualty of the pandemic. Nothing gold can stay, I suppose.) My first visit to the bridge was cut short by nightfall, but the next day I returned and resumed my search. After a couple of hours, I came upon the lock. I squealed in delight and immediately phoned Polina back in the United States to share with her my discovery, too excited to stop and check whether I would be rousing her from sleep.

The lock had survived the years and so had I, though my skating at Merkur Ice Stadium—the same place where we had trained in 2014—looked just as rusty. I finished ninth, one spot behind my U.S. teammate Clare Seo, who is eleven years my junior and was making her international senior debut.

I debated withdrawing from the 2023 U.S. Championships in San Jose. My injury had hampered my preparation for *months*. I couldn't train the way I wanted to. I could skate only four days a week, unable to do more than five reps of each jump per session. I discontinued my off-ice training to protect my hip. I felt like I was getting weaker and in more pain than ever. It's defeating to go into any competition knowing that you're not physically capable of performing your best. I began to wonder if my coaches were losing patience with me. I got the feeling that they believed my problem was more mental than physical. They kept pushing me to see a new clinical psychologist, and when I declined, they invited one to the rink—whom I refused to see. My pain was *real*. It was not in my head. I was not making it up to give myself a convenient excuse if I didn't achieve my goal, which I had been bold enough to declare out loud to reporters, of making the podium at nationals.

In the end, I decided to compete in San Jose because I was playing the long game. I was leaning toward extending my career at least another year, and if I did that, I would need a result from nationals or I'd be starting from scratch when it came to qualifying for the 2024 event.

I managed the short program well enough to make it into the final grouping for the free skate. I delivered my first positively graded triple-triple combination at a U.S. Championships since 2017 despite skating cautiously and babying my right hip. I stood only one and a half points out of third place going into the free skate, which was pretty incredible given my truncated training.

My eighth-place finish overall was my best showing at a nationals post-recovery. As soon as I turned my phone on after my free skate, I sent a text to Carly and my mom, who had departed the arena right after I left the ice: "I'm sorry, guys."

Why did I feel the need to apologize? Maybe I was overreacting, but I picked up on subliminal messages that made me wonder if some people thought I had overstayed my welcome in the sport. Not from the fans, who showered me with a standing ovation in San Jose and have been wildly supportive throughout my comeback. But from everyone else: the judges, who scored my short program awfully *conservatively;* the media, who mostly wrote up the women's short program without mentioning my placement, despite the fact that I was the only two-time national champion entered on the women's side; and U.S. Figure Skating, whose officials neglected to include me in the post-competition interview procession. It was a sobering reminder that youth *will* be served. My comeback had provided interesting copy for a year or two, but now everybody had moved on to the next big thing. In the star churn, I was one step away from completing the cycle of celebrity: Who is Gracie Gold? Yay, Gracie Gold! Who's the next Gracie Gold? Who was Gracie Gold?

It's sad that the best women in the world aren't staying in the sport until they become actual women. I'm thinking of Alysa Liu, who won her first U.S. title at thirteen and was out of the sport by her seventeenth birthday.

The reception I've received from the public suggests to me that those in charge of skating's promotion underestimate the appeal of grit and maturity. Consider my 2014 Olympic teammate Mikaela Shiffrin, the alpine skier who continues to rack up victories on the World Cup skiing circuit at twenty-seven (and shows no signs of slowing). Then there's the veteran track star Allyson Felix, who won a bronze medal at the Tokyo Olympics at the age of thirty-five. Why should skating be so different? If their examples are any indication, I have miles and miles to go on the ice. Can I land a triple Axel or a quad before I quit? Who knows, but I'm motivated to find out.

Throughout the 2022–23 season, I fielded questions from several fans who wondered if I would be participating in the Stars on Ice tour in the spring of 2023. They said they were hoping I'd be part of the cast because they'd gladly pay to watch me skate. How flattering that they think I have a say in the matter. I didn't have the heart to tell them that I'd never be considered for the show because my results don't qualify me as a "star." If I wanted to travel around the country to perform, it wouldn't be with the Stars on Ice tour.

The day after my free skate in San Jose, I received a text from an unfamiliar Colorado Springs–based number informing me that I was the third alternate for an international assignment. I thought it was a joke. I had been lucky to complete two programs on my bad hip. "LOL," I replied. My flippant response earned me a reprimand from U.S. Figure Skating because the text was real and had been sent by someone inside the organization. Whoops. I further alienated governing body officials when I was asked if I'd like to skate (for free, natch) in the exhibition at the conclusion of nationals and I responded that I would prefer not to.

The national governing body can't have it both ways. If I'm too old and washed up to cycle through the media mixed zone after I compete, fine, but then don't turn to me to help sell tickets for the nationals' final session, which is essentially why the exhibition exists. I thought about all the exhibitions I'd dutifully participated in where I was one of the few non-medalists, which always made me feel self-conscious, like the only wedding party member without a date. No, thank you. I don't think I'll do another. If the goal of these exhibitions was to excite young people about skating, there were other ways I could support the cause—and I would. But I was drawing my boundaries on the ice. Finally. And it felt good.

I left California feeling like I have nothing left to prove, but I still have a lot to give.

26

A SAFE SPACE TO SHARE

In treatment, it was impressed upon us that exercise is a great mood enhancer because physical activity releases chemicals that promote feelings of euphoria. Well, there's exercise, and then there's seven hours of grueling physical activity a day, six days a week, year in and year out for the better part of a decade. That's high-pressure, stressful *exertion*, which floods your system with the stress hormone cortisol. It's responsible for your body's fight-or-flight response, and too much of it coursing through your body over time can contribute to all kinds of health issues. I liken those of us in elite sports to squirrels that get zapped over and over on the electric fence that offers their only access to acorns. As I look toward my future, I want to be a mental health guide for those chasing greatness. I want to pass on the lessons that would have saved me.

As I consider my life after retirement, I'm reminded of a quote that I stumbled upon online: *We develop the character traits that would have saved our parents.* I think that's 100 percent accurate, and it's just as true if you substitute "coaches" for "parents."

In my "Road to Gold" clinics, my goal is to be the mentor I could have benefited from having when I was younger. What concrete shape my work with skaters takes remains to be seen. I have yet to figure it out. While at the United States Olympic and Paralympic Training Center rehabbing my left foot and right hip injuries, I met with Tracy Marek, the head of U.S. Figure Skating (and the first female chief executive of the organization in its 101-year history). Tracy is a longtime sports executive whose prior job was in marketing with the NBA's Cleveland Cavaliers. She doesn't have a skating background, which I consider a plus. She's bringing to the sport a wealth of management experience and a fresh outlook.

She invited me to her office in Colorado Springs. It was the first time I had been invited to the chief executive's office. She said she wanted to pick my brain. It was the first time the CEO of the federation had expressed an interest in hearing what I had to say. The meeting lasted two hours. Tracy took notes as I talked. Another first. I left her office feeling as if I had been truly heard by someone in U.S. Figure Skating. And not just anyone, but the boss. It gave me hope for the future.

Mental health was a major focus of our discussion. Based on my experience, I told her, every U.S. Figure Skating national team member should be handed a single-spaced sheet listing the side effects that they can expect to experience in their ascent: eating disorders, depression, anxiety, suicidal ideation.

I told her we have to have these hard conversations because there *still* is a stigma attached to mental illness, and that will continue to be the case as long as there are high achievers who are rewarded from an early age for pushing through their pain and "toughing it out."

It's not just a sports problem.

In October 2022, on my way to Skate America, I made a side

trip to New York to accept an award from the National Eating Disorders Association (NEDA). I have to admit. I was dubious at first. *Am I being recognized for being the best anorexic?*

It turned out to be one of the most amazing honors I've ever received. The awards gala was held at the Ziegfeld Ballroom, an art deco space in midtown that oozed New York glamour. In the same place seven months later, Meghan Markle, Duchess of Sussex, would receive a Woman of Vision award from Gloria Steinem.

During the cocktail hour, giant video boards strategically placed around the room flashed sobering statistics: Every fifty-two minutes, someone dies as a direct result of an eating disorder. Up to 45 percent of female athletes and 19 percent of male athletes struggle with an eating disorder (based on what I've observed, I'd say that both figures are considerably higher). Only 20 percent of medical schools offer elective training in eating disorders.

The evening's theme was "See the change. Be the change." Here was an organization obviously doing angels' work. To be recognized as somebody making a positive difference *off* the ice made me stand a little taller in my Rent the Runway dress.

At the head table I sat surrounded by impeccably clothed, impressively credentialed donors. Between courses, a woman leaned over and, in hushed tones, described the helplessness she had experienced when her daughter was in the grip of anorexia. *Keep doing what you're doing,* she said. *It's important.*

I know. I hear echoes of her words everywhere. I am transported to an ice show in Chicagoland, near the end of my 2022 touring schedule. I felt run down, worn out, exhausted. I was dead on my feet. During the meet-and-greet, a young woman I'll call Alice shyly slipped a note into my hand, then disappeared into the crowd. I didn't have a chance to read what she wrote until I was back in my hotel room.

> I just wanted to write this in case I never got the chance to say it—you are my biggest inspiration. In October of 2020, I spent three months at The Meadows Ranch among a few other facilities, and my mother told me about how you'd gone through the same thing. I thought I'd never skate again. Watching you bounce back with such beauty and grace has given me the hope nobody else could seem to provide. All thanks to you, I've been out of the hospital since April, back on the ice since June 2021. I came back with no jumps, but now I'm working on triples again. Thank you for pretty much saving my life by reigniting my passion for skating and giving me something to be well for again.

It was so moving. What better evidence do I need that I'm well on my way to being the change I wanted to see in the skating world? When I was in treatment and pondering my next course of action, I mapped out my future in my journal. I wrote that I would skate one more season, retire before I turned twenty-four, and enroll in medical school to study pediatrics, ophthalmology, family medicine, or oncology. Why those professions? Because "I can change lives," I wrote.

The intervening years have offered ample evidence that I don't need a fancy degree. I don't require another national title or an individual Olympic medal. Alice's beautiful note affirmed that everything I need to make a difference, I already possess.

At one of my clinics, a young girl raised her hand and asked, "Why did you stop eating?" It was a great question. I was impressed by her directness. Plenty of adults have wondered the same thing only to beat around the bush with a vague, *What happened to you?*

I mean, how much time do you have?

The question deserved an equally direct answer. I explained that I went through a period where a lot of stuff was happening in my life that was beyond my grasp and way beyond my ability to change or fix. I felt lost and lonely and confused and sad, and I didn't know what to do. I stopped eating because the amount of food I put in my mouth was the single thing I could control. I hurt myself before anybody else could. It's a messed-up form of autonomy, but for someone who felt isolated from her family and out of touch with her authentic self, my mental health issues became familiar and comfortable companions. It might have been too adult for a child's ears, but it was one of the more real and honest answers I could have given her.

In my appearances to talk about mental health, I make clear that there's no checklist, no official list of symptoms where if five or more describe you then you should seek immediate help. Things don't have to reach a specific threshold of pain before you are legitimately sick.

And something I can't emphasize enough, since I was guilty of this kind of martyr-complex thinking: *You don't get any medals for suffering in silence the longest.*

After stuffing down my feelings for so long to be palatable to the skating public, I continue to marvel at how I'm celebrated for speaking up. Especially when what I'm saying can make people uncomfortable. I wasted too many years and too much energy making myself small and pliable—unthreatening—because skating, like society, generally loves women who are quiet and easygoing and acquiescent. Women who don't make others squirm. If I seemed like vanilla before, I'm pistachio now. I always was full of texture and bursting with color, but vanilla was more palatable for the skating crowd. To my delight, I'm discovering that a surprising number of people are wild about pistachio.

In the fall of 2022, I also was honored at the Bell of Hope Celebration in downtown Philadelphia. I received a gorgeous, hefty bronze bell trophy from the Mental Health Partnerships in recognition of my personal resilience and public efforts to demystify mental health conditions. Another cocktail reception, another sad story. A woman told me her nine-year-old son used to be obsessed about figure skating. Then one day the coach with whom he had developed a strong rapport failed to show up for a scheduled session. She had died by suicide the night before. *I'm so sorry*, I said. I stayed by her side in case there was more she wanted to share. I'm not a trained mental health professional. I have no answers. But I have ears. I can listen. I can make sure people know that they are seen and heard.

That's something.

I sat down on a dais next to the master of ceremonies, who cued a two-minute clip of a 2020 interview I had done with the basketball star Chamique Holdsclaw, who also has suffered from depression.

The clip faded to black, and I was invited to speak. The first words out of my mouth were an apology. I told the audience that the interview they'd just seen had been me at my stammering, stumbling worst, in which I had struggled to string sentences together. "Hopefully," I said, "I'll be more eloquent this evening."

My friends in the audience squirmed in their seats. They exchanged knowing glances. I was perfectly eloquent in their eyes. I had no reason to apologize. But that's skating's fun-house mirror for you. We're constantly being judged on and off the ice. So why should anyone be surprised if I'm always looking at myself through a distorted lens?

At my "Road to Gold" seminars, we learned through trial and

error to hold the meet-and-greets first, then get down to the skating. Most of the kids at the places we visit have never met anybody they've seen on TV. At our first few clinics, they froze on the ice and stared at me instead of showing me their skills. If I meet them first, they quickly see that I'm just an ordinary person, allowing them to relax so we can get down to skating.

There's so much artifice in skating, but not at my seminars. I'm real with them. I tell the kids and their parents that if making it to the Olympics is the only reason they're in the sport, stop now, before the sacrifices and expenses pile up. I tell the kids that statistically they are more likely to be struck by lightning than compete in the Olympics.

Was my family intense on all fronts? Without question. Did my parents always set the bar high and expect Carly and me to clear it with room to spare? For sure. But my parents didn't push me into skating. I did it because I loved it.

If "just" making the national team or competing at nationals or mastering a double Axel had been as far as I got, it would have been a worthy pursuit in my parents' eyes. In the end, it was me, not my parents or Carly, who was never satisfied, who kept pushing, who lost sight of reality and turned skating into *The Hunger Games*. No one gets to the top in anything—school, work, sports—without sacrifices that might look a little excessive from the outside. Sometimes even from the inside. If it gets too intense, it's okay to adjust course. That's one lesson I wish had been drilled into me. Then again, if it had, I probably wouldn't be so gung ho about passing on what I know now to the next generation.

27

CALL ME COACH

I'll never forget the day that Vinnie, a baby-faced teenager, landed his first double loop in competition as part of a free skate that featured four passes with double jumps, another first.

At that point, I had been coaching Vinnie for more than four years. An Olympic cycle and then some. I knew that program was a long time in the making, and when it came to fruition it was a toss-up as to which of us was more thrilled. Those breakthrough moments when students push through their fears and insecurities, give gravity the middle finger, and soar fill me with joy.

I'm sure none of the men or women who went bald or gray working with me imagined that I'd follow them into coaching. The fact is, few of skating's highest achievers stick around in the sport once their competitive careers are over unless it's to provide TV commentary. The last U.S. Olympic medalist in ladies' singles to devote herself full-time to coaching that I'm aware of was Carol Heiss Jenkins, and she retired from competitive skating in 1960.

A conversation with a two-time Olympian, a contemporary of mine, was instructive in understanding why so few since have followed Carol's example. This skater expressed bewilderment that I had chosen to coach. In her mind, there could be only one explanation. "Oh, so you don't have anything else to do?" she asked.

Au contraire, I told her. I've seen a lot of the world beyond skating, enough of it, anyway, to know there's nowhere I'd rather be than on the ice.

I have serious doubts about whether I'm cut out to be a mother, but the longer I coach the surer I am that I'm meant to guide children. I have a soft spot for them, even the little girl at one of my clinics who declared, "You have a voice that makes you sound unintelligent." Oh my God, how can you not applaud her directness?

I love kids because they don't bullshit you. I love skating because it's the spoonful of honey that makes the life lessons go down easier. To be able to teach skating to kids (and adults who are young at heart) is, for me, pretty much the perfect marriage of passion and purpose.

I wish I could say that I choreographed this career move, but the truth is I sort of stumbled into coaching. I emerged from treatment needing to work, for the daily structure it provided as much as for the paycheck. When I started teaching lessons at a rink in Scottsdale, Arizona, I was not at all certain that it would be something I'd be any good at.

The better an athlete is at their craft, the worse they generally are at teaching it, which doesn't surprise me in the least. So much of what separates the best athletes from the rest is hard to quantify and harder to explain. How do you teach feel and instinct and desire and obsession?

My own coaching learning curve was steep. How did I translate skills that have become second nature in a way that others could easily understand? It took me forever to figure out how to coach a Lutz, for example, because the outside-edge takeoff that gives a lot of people fits came naturally to me.

No one seemed bothered by my inexperience. What mattered was I was still Gracie Gold, Olympian and two-time national champion. My CV preceded me through the door at Scottsdale's Ice Den (and the location in nearby Chandler, where I also worked on occasion). People didn't care if I could coach or not. They considered it worth the price of a lesson for themselves or their darlings to share the ice with a real live Olympic medalist. They could learn sit spins for $90 and get a selfie with me for free.

In the beginning, I considered coaching nothing more than a step sequence, a bridge from recovery to my next move, which I assumed would be training for a career in something *important* like medicine.

Skating entered the chat.

One day I choreographed an actual step sequence for a skater and watched with growing annoyance as she made a complete hash of it. I decided to demonstrate it for her, in the spirit of *I'm a cow on skates and I can do this, so there's absolutely no reason why you can't, too.* I had no idea anybody was watching until several other skaters and coaches started clapping when I finished. I felt mildly embarrassed but mostly exhilarated. I have and always will love to skate and perform. That love had been dormant for a long time until the applause awakened it.

Before long, a seed of a mission statement took root in my mind: What if I could pass on to my students the beauty of skating without inflicting the pain that I had endured? I stuck a pin in that thought and got on with my twelve-hour days. As the new person at the rink, I was funneled some of the so-called head cases and untalented students and realized they were some of my favorite people to work with. I recognized a bit of myself in each of them, if I'm honest. If they required a little extra effort on my part, well, it was no more than my coaches had lavished on me.

After two months I moved to the rink in suburban Philadelphia, lured there in part by the promise of more coaching opportunities. Vinnie became one of my first students. He didn't say a lot at first, but over the years I've watched him emerge from his shell as a human being and skater. His breakthrough program was still a few months on the horizon when his mom texted me about Vinnie:

> In the few years we have known you, you have been such a role model and positive influence on him. The changes on the outside everyone can see as he gets taller and older, but you have helped shape the changes on the inside and for that I could not be more grateful. Thank you for being his hero.

I'm not ugly crying! You're ugly crying. And speaking of tears . . . In 2021, Vinnie struggled through a mistake-marred program at a competition in New York City and was sobbing so hard he was practically dry heaving on the bench near the front door, in full view of everybody in Chelsea Piers' fishbowl rink.

He had told his mother after a mistake-marred warmup that he wanted to withdraw. "That's not how it works," I said. I explained that I've lost count of the number of times I wanted to quit after a crime scene of a short program. But one of the first lessons you learn in skating is to honor a commitment, be it a forty-minute session on the ice or a weekend competition.

I've worked with kids, including Vinnie on occasion, who can't wait to be done with the lessons their parents have paid for. After five minutes, they're not listening to a word I say. *It's okay if skating isn't your jam,* I tell them. *I understand if you don't want to be here. Some days neither do I. But somebody has paid for you to be on the ice with me right now, so let's pick one thing that we could try to make a little better and focus on that.*

Vinnie's training in the lead-up to the New York City juvenile event had not gone well, to say the least. He had been battling a hip injury and seemed so unprepared that I suggested he forgo the competition. I suspected that if he did skate and struggled, as I was almost certain he would, his mental health would suffer. But he said he really wanted to get another competition under his belt before regionals. (I recognize now how similar his stubbornness was to my own in the lead-up to my Rostelecom Cup debacle, and I think a lot about how I can better use my experiences to coach in moments like these going forward. If I had to do it over, I'd have put my foot down and insisted that he stay home. Live and learn.) He said he didn't care how it went. But obviously he did.

We were seated maybe five feet away from the boards, and it was pin-drop silent in the rink except for his sobbing. All eyes were either on him or actively avoiding him. I thought it was self-indulgent and immature to draw attention to himself like that. Whether he realized it or not, he was detracting from the experience of the next competitor.

I ushered him to a back corner of the lobby, where we could have a modicum of privacy. And then—and I want to preface this by saying it wasn't my proudest moment—I said, "Do you think you're the only one who didn't skate up to their expectations today? You think you're the only one who has been devastated by how they performed? You don't cause a scene while another kid is getting ready to skate. You cry in the bathroom like everyone else and don't come out until you're done!"

That last remark apparently made an impression on Vinnie. While out with his mom one day not long thereafter, he watched her step in mud that splattered all over her clothes and practically swallowed her ankles. She got upset, and Vinnie, with the sweetest of smiles, I'm told, said, "In the wise words of Gracie Gold, go cry in the bathroom like everyone else and don't come out until you're done!"

I laughed out loud when Vinnie's mom relayed that story. Working with kids really does give me *fou de joie*. Mad joy. Three weeks after he landed all those doubles in competition for the first time, Vinnie had a bad day at practice. He kept falling on his double Salchow–double loop combination. He was visibly frustrated. But he didn't give up. Something had clicked. He was mad because he knew he was capable of landing those jumps, not because he didn't think he ever would. I turned my back so he wouldn't see me smiling.

I'm a pretty good teacher. But you know who's the best teacher? Failure. Some of my greatest epiphanies have occurred in the split second before my ass hits the ice. It's what I tell my students all the time. If we're so afraid of failure that we don't try, how will we ever improve as skaters and grow as people?

I've fallen a hundred thousand times in my skating career. And that's probably a conservative estimate. So when a student describes themselves as "garbage" after falling twice, my reflexive response is, "What does that make me? The city dump?" I don't know when, where, or why, but falling has gotten a bad rap. I've spent fifteen minutes of an Axel class watching a dozen kids remain upright, and I'm here to tell you, that's just not okay.

I tell my students all the time that nothing impedes success like the fear of failure. If you don't fall during a thirty-minute lesson, I'm sorry, but that doesn't impress me much.

I've come across kids in my clinic who expect to be praised if they stay on their feet, even if their mechanics are terrible. That's not going to happen on my watch. I had a mother get in my face and yell, "Why did you tell my daughter she isn't trying and she'll never get her Axel?" I calmly explained that in a forty-five-minute session, her daughter had not fallen once, nor had she made any alterations to improve her technique, presumably because of a fear of falling. "It's fine to live life in your comfort zone," I said, "but only if you adjust your expectations on what will be accomplished."

I tell my students that the real failure occurs when they're so afraid to mess up that they don't make an effort. I've been known to stop an Axel class and say, "Nobody's falling, which means nobody's trying." Mistakes are a part of learning. If I am here to teach them something new, I remind them, why do they expect that they'll be proficient by the end of the session?

I also tell my students that anyone who shames them for falling, especially when learning a jump, is someone to be tuned out. If that someone is a parent, let the coach set them straight, kindly but firmly. If it's a coach, they're not the one for you.

I see my job as helping students reach their equivalent of the Olympics, whatever that looks like. Maybe it's executing a clean Axel or a double combination. Maybe it's qualifying for the U.S. Adult Figure Skating Championships. Maybe it's living life outside their comfort zone. I reject the belief, all too prevalent in the sport, that if you're not on an Olympic track there's no path for you.

Coaching has given me so much. It has made me a better athlete. If my students are watching, I know that I *have* to finish a terrible run-through because it's what I lecture them to do every week. After I eat shit on a jump, I know I need to pop up and immediately do another jump to show that falls are no big deal and to demonstrate fearlessness.

Let me be clear. I totally don't want to do any of these things. But I also don't want to be a hypocrite. That means practicing what I preach.

Coaching has improved my mental health. When I'm in a bad headspace, if I can turn around and help a student with a spin, jump, or step sequence, I instantly feel better. Every. Single. Time.

And at the start of my comeback, when I was moving on the ice like a potato on skates, the adults I was coaching—including a seventy-seven-year-old man who enjoys competing in a way I can only aspire to—helped me get my mojo back. I'd watch their lack of self-consciousness and eagerness to try new skills, and it inspired me to become the best version of my current self—and not the old Gracie.

In the six years I've been coaching, that seed of a mission statement that took root in my mind—teaching what is beautiful about skating without inflicting the pain that I endured—has grown and flourished. I have so many ideas for how to save skating from the perils that have been a blight on its beauty. Here's where I'd start, with the establishment of a hotline that would place experts in various fields at coaches' fingertips.

A male coach who doesn't know how to deal with a teenage girl in the throes of puberty? There'd be a child development psychologist on call to advise him. A coach with a skater who appears to have a problematic relationship with food? Contact this vetted disordered-eating expert. A coach with a skater struggling with their sexuality? Here's a trained counselor with suggestions on how they can best support their athlete. The hotline would address three incontrovertible truths: Everyone needs help sometimes. No one has all the answers. Too few people even have the right questions.

I want to be the change that skating needs, which is why I set aside time at each "Road to Gold" clinic for Q&As with small groups of skaters. The parents are forewarned that I won't shy away from sensitive topics, so if they or their children have any qualms about my not sticking to skating, they are welcome to skip over this part of the schedule.

After the inaugural clinic, we solicited feedback from the parents of the children who attended. Did they find the question-and-answer session beneficial? More than one parent reached out to say their kids came home and proceeded to open up for the first time about problems or struggles they were having.

I'm headed in the right direction. I just have to keep putting one skate in front of the other.

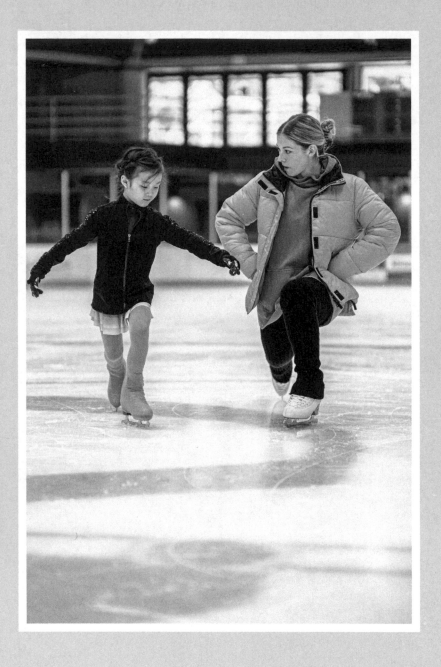

EPILOGUE

Spring 2023 finds me holed up in another dorm every inch as charmless as my accommodations at The Meadows were nearly six years ago. I'm at the Olympic Training Center in Colorado Springs for several weeks of treatment of a different kind, this time for a broken left foot. For two months I've been hobbling around in a knee-length boot. My days pass in a monotonous loop of physical therapy appointments, for both my foot and my right hip, which still is bothering me and so far has eluded a diagnosis. The forced inactivity has given me ample time to ponder my future—and whether it will or should include competitive skating.

Twice a week I've been catching a ride to the Sertich Ice Center to coach an old friend at the morning adult session. It's illuminating and inspiring to watch people from all walks of life practice the sport I grew up doing. They aren't skating for medals or pursuing Olympic dreams. They don't care that skating is a sport where a twenty-seven-year-old is considered ancient. They're there because they love it. After one such trip to the rink, I re-

turned to my dorm room and, sprawled on the twin bed, tapped
out another letter.

July 2023

Dear Skating,

*The last time I wrote to you I was in the middle of the godfor-
saken desert, surrounded by self-help quotes, therapists, and
scorpions. I was thrumming with sadness, resentment, and Prozac. I'll be the first to admit that my last letter to you was a
touch dramatic. But then, it was a Dear John letter signifying the
end of my longest-lasting relationship I've had outside of my immediate family.*

*You were my first love. Our relationship has been a tumultu-
ous one. You are the second-greatest gift life has bestowed upon
me, after my twin sister. People often ask, "If you weren't a skater,
what would you be?" I've always hated that question, because
I've always considered myself SO much more than a skater. It just
took me a long time to recognize that. But there's no denying that
it's because of you that I've seen parts of the world I never expected to visit and met parts of me that I never knew were there.*

*Not to sound like a dime-store novel cliché, but it's not you.
It's me. You were never the problem. Previously, I said that you
brought me to the highest highs and the lowest lows. But in the
six years since I wrote that, I've come to realize that I brought
myself to those places. The gifts and the failures were my own
handiwork, no one else's. But why blame myself when I could
point the finger elsewhere?*

*Your culture can be elitist and judgmental. There are so many
unspoken rules, and the politics are more complex than on Capi-*

tol Hill. I struggled in your misogynistic and anachronistic world to be my true self. So I settled on being someone else, someone who I thought everyone would like. I became Gracie Gold, the completely unrelatable and entirely predictable ice princess. I thought you would love me more if I changed myself, but I really hated who I became. I blamed you for my pain, my identity crisis, my family's collapse, my lost childhood.

From my vantage point now, I clearly see it was everything around you that was to blame: the federation, the coaches, the culture, the judges, and the media. They were the toxins, not you, because you, skating, are amazing.

"Why did you come back to skating?" Everybody has asked me that question, and it's hard not to read between the lines and conclude that people think you're no good for me. That I should have stayed away from you. That I could do so much better. But as I see it, they're asking the wrong question. It should be, "Why did you ever leave?" And if I was asked that, I'd say, simply, because I had lost my faith that you and I could bring out the best, not the worst, in each other. I came back after deciding to trust that you could help me heal and grow and get better. That you could help me spread the word that age is but a number, that skills and confidence are never really lost; they just sometimes go dormant or atrophy from underuse.

So many people leave you bitter and resentful. Regretful that they entrusted their hearts and souls to you. Six years ago, I was well on my way to becoming one of them. I'm so grateful that I saw the wrongheadedness of my thinking before it was too late. Because now I see your intrinsic beauty and the gifts you freely give to enrich the lives of so many all over the world. I have you to thank for showing me how resilient I can be. How athletic. How confident, driven, hard-working, kind, and brave. Without question, the best moments in my life have been with you, right alongside some of the worst.

All of this is to say I'm sorry. I'm sorry that the culture around you is so toxic. That the most unstable, most unwell people seem to be drawn to your orbit like planets to the sun. I'm sorry that so many athletes, including myself for a spell, hobble away from you broken and resentful. Most of all, I'm sorry that it took leaving you for me to realize how much I love you. I could have loved you differently, but I could not have loved you more.

I don't care what anybody says. I'm so thankful to be back in your arms. Thank you for being the biggest facet in the rough-cut diamond that is me.

All my love,

GG

ACKNOWLEDGMENTS

Working on this memoir has given me the opportunity to look back on my life with a new sense of clarity and gratitude. Here are a few special people to whom I'd like to extend my particular thanks:

To Carly for being the Artemis to my Nike, the sunshine to my storm cloud, and for being the better half. I wouldn't have gone on this journey without you, nor would I have wanted to. Thank you for being my best friend.

To my mom for her undying belief that I could and would do great things in this world. Thank you for all the sacrifices you made along the way.

To James for loving me even when I am entirely unlovable. Thank you for being the kindest, most empathetic, and most supportive man I have ever met.

To Pasha for your time and your patience and for being the father/brother I never had growing up. I stumbled into your life at rock bottom. You and Alex held my hand as I found my feet and the ice again. I will never be able to repay you two for giving me a second chance.

To my close friends, including Tara for being my biggest advocate, for sharing the paychecks and amazing experiences, and for helping me write the memoir I always wanted; Shannon for being instrumental in the process of writing this book; Kelsey for the endless conversations, support, and the Monacos; Leif for metaphorically holding my hand; Michael D. for loving and supporting Carly; Mirai and Michael B. for the humor and honesty; Craig for the unwavering support and unforgettable times; Peter for your knowledge and help; Amy for keeping Road 2 Gold and me together even when I was falling apart; and Jeremy for your humor, creativity, and genuine friendship.

To my former training mates and friends in skating for inspiring me, wiping my tears, encouraging me, and offering camaraderie in this wild sport.

To the figure-skating fans who have stood by me and cheered me on throughout my career, and to the people who have shared their stories of surviving skating, mental illness, eating disorders, and more with me on the road. Thank you for your generosity, which has made me feel supported and seen.

To my students, like Vinnie (my first and favorite student), for challenging me to be a better coach and a better role model; to Tammy, Beth, and Kevin for reminding me that skating looks good on all ages; to Sou for truly being my number one fan.

To my mentors, like Amy and Max, for my start on the ice; Cruella for showing me what kind of coach I don't want to be; Toni for the encouragement and patience; Alex O. for the technique and belief in me; Frank for the wisdom, stability, and guidance; Marina and Oleg for taking me in at my lowest point; Lori for the inspiration and the beautiful programs; Michael S. for the support, laughs, and love; Rockne for standing with me at that one Champs Camp when no one else would; and Jenny Convisor for holding me, my career, and my family together, and for inspiring us to be brave even in our darkest times.

To Lorrie Parker for being an unstoppable force of positivity, light, and patriotism; J for your transparency, candor, stability, and leadership; Mia for making me laugh and being a good human; Ingrid for answering every single email and text we sent you; Angelita for booking every flight and handling every travel crisis.

To the staff, techs, and other patients at The Meadows for saving my life and helping me put my pieces back together.

To Karen Crouse for going on this journey with me and helping me write a better memoir than I could have ever dreamed possible.

To Mia Vitale and Sarah Passick at Park Fine Literary for helping my memoir dreams come true, and for finding me the perfect home.

To Matt Inman for the edits and the guidance, which helped me craft my story, and to the team at Crown, including Stacey Stein and Julie Cepler, for helping me share it with the world.

PHOTO CREDITS

ABOUT THE AUTHOR

GRACIE GOLD is a two-time U.S. figure skating champion and Olympic bronze medalist. She is the first and only American woman to win an NHK Trophy title and holds the record for the highest short program score ever recorded by an American woman. Her writing has been published in *The Cut*. She lives in Wilmington, Delaware, and trains in suburban Philadelphia.

ABOUT THE TYPE

This book was set in Minion, a 1990 Adobe Originals typeface by Robert Slimbach. Minion is inspired by classical, old-style typefaces of the late Renaissance, a period of elegant and beautiful type designs. Created primarily for text setting, Minion combines the aesthetic and functional qualities that make text type highly readable with the versatility of digital technology.